ADOLESCENT PSYCHIATRY

DEVELOPMENTAL AND CLINICAL STUDIES

VOLUME XI

Annals of the American Society for Adolescent Psychiatry

ADOLESCENT PSYCHIATRY

DEVELOPMENTAL AND CLINICAL STUDIES

VOLUME XI

Edited by

MAX SUGAR
Editor in Chief

Senior Editors
SHERMAN C. FEINSTEIN
JOHN G. LOONEY
ALLAN Z. SCHWARTZBERG
ARTHUR D. SOROSKY

The University of Chicago Press
Chicago and London

The University of Chicago Press, Chicago 60637
The University of Chicago Press, Ltd., London

International Standard Book Number: 0-226-77962-9
Library of Congress Catalog Card Number: 70-147017

CONTENTS

PREFACE

After ten years of superb leadership by the founding editors of *Adolescent Psychiatry,* the Annals of the American Society for Adolescent Psychiatry, the mantle of responsibility has now been shifted. I hope to fulfill the editorial task as I learn to navigate in these new waters. I further hope to emulate my predecessors and to provide you, the readers, with an annual volume that will be welcomed as a valuable addition to your clinical and theoretical work with adolescents.

We note and mourn the death of Anna Freud on October 8, 1982. This brilliant, dedicated pioneer in child and adult psychoanalysis has given us a beacon, built on her exemplary observations and theory. We dedicate this volume to her memory.

MAX SUGAR

EDITOR'S INTRODUCTION

Despite a change of editors, the general editorial objective remains that initiated by my predecessors: for *Adolescent Psychiatry* to be a superb, scholarly volume. In this endeavor, we plan to explore adolescence as a process and to publish work on the clinical and developmental aspects of adolescence. Adolescent psychiatry has matured, deepened, and broadened in recent decades; thus one goal will be to keep up with changes in the field and present new theories and data on adolescence.

This first volume of *Adolescent Psychiatry*'s second decade demonstrates these concerns and aspirations, for it covers theoretical, technical, and clinical issues from a psychoanalytic view; therapeutic problems with special groups; cultural and research aspects of the family of the adolescent; the *Umwelt* of adolescents with sensory deprivation; and the problem of learning deficits in college.

The volume opens with a memorial to Anna Freud written by one of her many students, colleagues, friends, and admirers, Rudolf Ekstein.

Reflecting on the relationship of adolescence and parenthood, Erik H. Erikson focuses on the importance of fidelity and care and reminds us of the special problems we face when these qualities are absent.

Albert J. Solnit provides us with a perspective on helps and hindrances in the transition from adolescence to parenthood. Parenthood requires completion of adolescent developmental tasks, a completion which enables a sense of confidence and competence to develop.

Many adolescents construct fantasy families. Sol Nichtern explores how such "families" affect the adolescent process and how they serve as vehicles for the transmission of values from one generation to another, thus affecting society at large.

David A. Rothstein develops a thesis on adolescents' use of violence to solve the identity crisis. The army, for example, fills an intrapsychic void by providing a structure and transmits social values unchanged. Rothstein notes the part violence plays in large social groups and proposes the existence of an interplay between violence on the individual and societal levels.

Reporting research findings on two groups of competent adolescents—one from black, working-class families and the other from white, middle-class families—John G. Looney and Jerry M. Lewis find that the family has a powerful effect on adolescent development.

Laurie M. Brandt views the fairy tale as a useful therapeutic device to understand and deal with borderline patients who read them. Knowing the tales' specific contents allows the therapist to understand some of the developmental conflicts and to use the tales metaphorically as models for their resolution.

Deborah Anne Sosin proposes that diaries in adolescence may be considered transitional objects since they mirror, soothe, and help integrate adolescents' inner and outer realities. The diary may be used in psychotherapy as another window to understand and help the adolescent.

The case of an adolescent girl and her phobic reaction is presented by Peter Blos and used as a vehicle for a discussion of psychoanalytic concepts and their application to the psychotherapy of adolescents. The therapy, theoretical concepts, and technical aspects are described briefly but with great clarity.

According to Rudolf Ekstein, termination of treatment with adolescents is a process itself. He discusses several cases and notes that, with adolescents, termination is dependent on development as well as conflict resolution. The end is thus a beginning, where treatment is a prologue to the future and its uncertainties.

Carl B. Feinstein reports observations on the profound effects of communication problems on the development and functioning of adolescent deaf boys. He looks particularly at problems in socializing due to the lack of a peer support group.

Michael H. Stone discusses therapy problems of the borderline patient from a wealthy family, whose fortune insulates the adolescent from reality. This leads to difficulties in self-discipline and identity formation in the disturbed "VIP" youngsters and calls for special considerations in their treatment.

The assessment and diagnosis of learning disabilities in the college youngster are described by Jonathan Cohen. He considers the importance of recognizing emotional and organic factors, as well as the possibilities for enhancing the education of learning disabled youth.

Therapists may regard their patients' stories of sexual abuse as fantasy. However, Max Sugar emphasizes the need to consider material about sexual abuse of youngsters as a traumatic fact that interferes with development and contributes to emotional conflict. The molested youngster has a strong likelihood of becoming the molester in a constellation of neglect and a pathological symbiosis.

1   AS I REMEMBER HER: ANNA FREUD, 1895–1982

RUDOLF EKSTEIN

In recent years, whenever I traveled to Europe, I visited the Hampstead Clinic, sometimes to present a paper and always, I hoped, to have a visit with Anna Freud. In her last year, 1982, I could not see her there because she was in the hospital. Later, when Anna Freud was at home, she let me know through her secretary that most likely I would be able to see her. But first I would give a paper at the Hampstead Clinic.

In previous years, Anna Freud would usually chair the meeting and open the discussion. I remember well my apprehension when I spoke about a difficult case in which I was not quite sure how to begin the first therapeutic session. My thoughts went back to former clinical teachers, such as Anna Freud and August Aichhorn, and it was Aichhorn's way that seemed to be the best in this case. Anna Freud smiled, and, in her discussion, she joined me in feeling that it was Aichhorn's way of working that seemed to be best for the youngster that I was to see.

But I also recall another meeting on a panel with her in Vienna, the very same year, addressing teachers on the relationship between psychoanalysis and education. It was the field of education that was her first interest and remained important to her, similar to my own development in our field. She could be critical but was always objective, polite, accepting, and helpful. She always spoke *ad rem* and never *ad hominem*. She made one aspire to do the very best. She always allowed and encouraged us to have our own thoughts and methods.

But this time, June 30, 1982, it was Dr. Hansi Kennedy who chaired the meeting and ably introduced the discussion. I looked around the room at all the competent teachers that Anna Freud had gathered around her through the years. They have made the Hampstead Child Therapy Clinic in London famous, a place to revisit and from which to gain strength. I spoke about the termination phase in the treatment of adolescents, and I learned much from the discussion which later enabled me to revise the paper.

After that meeting, I was to cross the street from Twenty-one Maresfield Garden to Twenty Maresfield Garden, Freud's home. My colleagues had prepared me for the visit, and I realized that my wife and I should stay but a very few minutes.

I found Anna Freud outside in the garden, resting on a couch as I knew her father did during his last months in 1939. Her body was frail, her speech not always clear, but the spirit was there as always. Up to the last, I know, she remained interested in our work, and she asked me about my experience in Vienna. I know that she kept in touch on a day-to-day basis with the events, the training, the treatment, and the research at the clinic across the street. But when my wife, Ruth, and I left, we both knew this would be the last visit, the last good-bye, not the usual *auf Wiedersehen*. In those painful moments, high points of the past years flew by.

It was in 1935, the fall of that year, that I heard her for the first time at the old Psychoanalytic Institute in Berggasse, a few houses away from Berggasse Nineteen, Freud's home, and today the Freud Museum. She came with Dorothy Burlingham, her lifelong friend and collaborator, and addressed those of us who were in training there to become Psychoanalytic Pedagogues. I had recently started this program which was to supplement my education at the University of Vienna. It soon became my professional core interest. Sometime in 1937, I was to start my own analysis. I recall those moments in the waiting room when I entered Berggasse Nineteen for the first time and was interviewed by Anna Freud.

The war years and the escape from Austria made us refugees. But even in London, under uncertain conditions, the work and the inspiration went on. I still have the admission ticket, number 140, which allowed me to hear the lectures and classes for teachers, offering "Three Lectures on Psychology by Miss A. Freud," the first to take place on October 27, 1938. We continued the seminars, and with them grew a stronger commitment to psychoanalysis which kept us together through all those years of fascism in Central Europe, of being a refugee, of the Second World War, and of the slow postwar rebuilding.

Beyond reading her first communications about the work she, Dorothy Burlingham, and their collaborators did for children who were orphans and victims of the war, my contact with her was limited. But a short time after the war, around 1948, our correspondence resumed. I was at the Menninger Foundation then and assembled a Freud Issue of the *Bulletin of the Menninger Clinic,* and Anna Freud contributed.

Later, we met at international conferences and at the Menninger Foundation. I recall an experience shared with my then adolescent daughter, Jean, now an experienced teacher, who was at that time thinking of becoming one. She heard Anna Freud then for the first time and wanted to find out whether my respect and fondness for Anna Freud were "exaggerated." Afterward, she told me, "Dad, now I know what you mean. She is a wonderful lecturer, a great teacher. But I think I knew all these things anyway." How difficult it was for her to understand that it was precisely Anna Freud's clear and beautiful language that made it possible for us to listen, understand her, and somehow feel that "we knew it anyway." That was the way she wrote and the way that I had often heard her address large audiences, summarizing and synthesizing scientific papers of a whole congress while making it all come alive for us. This made us wish we could achieve her clarity, creativity, and capacity to transport herself into the mind of the listener. She identified with us, and thus we could identify with her.

During one of my visits, I brought her little gifts from the children of the Anna Freud Kindergarten in Vienna and greetings from its teachers. I know how proud she was that the city which she was once forced to leave had named a kindergarten after her and had helped create a living bridge between the work in London and that in Vienna. I knew then how wounds can heal.

Late in December 1979, I had sent a condolence note to her when Dorothy Burlingham died. In her response she said, "You are quite right that the generation before you is now going out and yours will become the old one." In spite of her growing weakness and the repeated hospitalizations, up to the very end she answered every letter; many of her answers were written in her own hand, and only late this last year did she ask her secretary to write to me for her.

Once we had her nephew, Ernst Freud, as a guest in our home in Brentwood. I asked him, "How is Anna Freud?" He told me that he had asked her what she wanted to have conveyed to friends and colleagues. Anna Freud told him to say to us, "Wanderer, kommst du nach Sparta, sage, du habest uns hier liegen gesehen, wie das Gesetz es befahl!" ("Wanderer, if thou comest to Sparta, tell them you have seen us lying here as was ordered by the law.") She quoted a sentence that we all had learned by heart in our European high schools. Those were the words of Leonidas, defending the culture of Athens against the invading Persians. I suppose that, to the last, she thought of herself as defending psychoanalysis, the work of her father, maintaining it, enlarging on it, and living up to her inner law. In that sense she had become for us Antigone who continues to speak for us, as she spoke for her father, and to lead us through the darkness of the unconscious and to help us maintain the humanitarian and scientific tradition.

As we were leaving her, I thought of the tired body, and I thought of the colleagues at the Hampstead Clinic who must now carry on the work based on the memory of a good and loving Antigone, a name that Professor Freud once gave her. They are strong and good people, and they will continue. When I think of that and our own determination to help them and carry on the work here, the tired face of Anna Freud disappears. It is replaced by a smiling and friendly face, the beautiful face of younger years, along with her humor, her strength, and the powerful example she set for us. She was a person who dedicated her life to children, to parents, and to all of us who work with children, who had found meaning in her life and had given to so many of us a professional life of meaning and dedication. When I think of that I realize in some ways I am no longer lonely. That is the way I remember her!

2 REFLECTIONS

ERIK H. ERIKSON

I

It is a pleasure to focus on the theme of the relationship of adolescence and parenthood. This certainly shows a hospitable trend toward such theories of the life cycle as Joan Erikson and I first presented to the Midcentury White House Conference (Erikson and Erikson 1948). There, however, we listed, between adolescence and adulthood, a stage of young adulthood to which we assigned the solution of one of life's vital conflicts, that is, intimacy versus isolation—a solution which is decisive for the strength and quality of adult love. To adolescence we had ascribed the crisis of identity versus identity confusion, the solution of which helped to develop the lifelong strength of fidelity; while adulthood and parenthood were marked by the crisis of generativity versus stagnation and the emergence of the strength of care. Now, generativity, reminiscent as the word is both of genitality and of generation, encompasses procreativity as well as productivity and creativity.

I would not have exposed you, at the beginning of a short communication, to all these high-sounding terms if I did not need them all for the question I have chosen to reflect on for this occasion—namely, how does that stage of young adulthood mediate between adolescence and adulthood? This permits me, at any rate, for the most systematic reasons, but also, I am afraid, in a somewhat dogmatic and repetitious manner, to address the otherwise pleasant theme of the indispensability of *intimacy* and *love*.

II

In our scheme even the most positive quality of life, intimacy, which is the very medium of love, has a counterpart, the threat of isolation. That is one of those dystonic and painful tendencies without which no human being can develop. While this conflict is to be resolved in young adulthood, in adolescence states of being in love and feeling isolated can alternate dramatically. In fact, as clinicians we have become aware of the tendency of adolescent patients to flee from early love into isolation. A corresponding flight is noticeable in their hesitation to develop the positive transference on which analyzability depends. Instead, we observe a partial regression to that early stage of infancy where a sense of "I" must emerge from trustful interplay with the maternal figure. The fact is that intimate love as well as positive transference can begin to mature only *after* a sense of identity has developed to a point where it can be shared and counterpointed with the identities of age-mates and mentors: only then can the young individual experience the fact that to lose oneself in love can mean to find oneself.

III

In this young adult development is also to be found the link between the psychosexual and the psychosocial aspects of the adolescent process. For one cannot graduate from puberty in a truly genital manner without the readiness for mutuality, even as true intimacy cannot develop without a mutual commitment to a general give-and-take.

Here, incidentally, I can never omit mentioning a certain respectful sadness over the way in which a field like ours can become addicted to the use of simple terms, such as the "self-object" relationship where the "object" is a truly loved person. To Freud, of course, it was libido, the "love energy," which was seeking objects to "cathex," while the whole person in search of love needs other persons who can afford to reciprocate. This is, of course, what adolescents begin to look for in smaller and larger groupings in the pursuit of joint involvements. In other words, they seek to commit themselves to a solidarity which in a more or less ideological form will prove itself indispensable for all adulthood and, above all, for parenthood. Parenthood calls for an extension of the sense of identity to include a sense of "We." This should permit a procreative "familiarity" which makes it possible to jointly bring up "our kind."

IV

If we may say, then, that identity can be relatively secure only if shared within a system of intimacy, while intimacy depends on what one has learned to love to be and to do together, there is good reason to reserve the word "object" for the things in the thing world. In all of cultural history, things, when properly attended to, have provided a shared sense of beauty as well as a shared cognitive affirmation of the "objective" lawfulness governing natural matters as well as technological and scientific methods. This is a massive aspect of human life almost totally ignored in much of the theoretical preoccupation with the self (and as for the self itself, who points to it and affirms it if not the sense of I which presides over the pronominal core of all languages?).

V

Let me now reflect on two historical matters of vital concern.

The first relates to Nichtern's (1983) focus on the fantasy family under various modern conditions. It contains impressive statistics on the dramatic increase of the present number of families in this country (one is inclined to put this word in quotation marks) which have little or no resemblance to the traditional pattern of the biological, two-parent family. In psychoanalytic terms, one cannot help asking two questions arising from our (I think necessary) assumption that generativity in adulthood has a procreative core which represents a final stage of psychosexuality beyond that of genitality. Can we expect the rapidly increasing number of children dependent on adults who are not their biological parents but play parental roles in their lives to be brought up effectively? Another question concerns the (necessarily and optionally) increasing number of adults who may become parents of only one or two children. What will happen to their, maybe, much more ambitious procreative inclinations or identifications? Clinical reports, no doubt, will throw light on pathological outcomes in both these cases. Positive impressions, however, may well indicate what could be of great importance for the future of mankind, namely, that generative drives can be—besides being used for productive purposes—in principle applied to all the children under one's immediate care (such as one's mate's children) or, indeed, to all children for whom one can learn to feel responsible. And, of course, the planned reduction of the number of children and the growing variety of familial patterns in the modern world coincide with this century's new insights into the nature and function of childhood.

VI

But just as we seem to be potentially closer to a living concept of a family of man, we face—or, rather, we suddenly realize that we have failed to face—the fact that all the children now alive or to be born in this world are living under a sinister cloud of extinction. This corresponds to what Robert Lifton (1974) has called "technicism"—a belief that any expansion of technical know-how is praiseworthy and guiltless, even if it is dangerous to other human beings, as long as we can project on them certain hostile attitudes. This I must, in conclusion, briefly relate to the stages of life.

Each of the three stages under discussion in these reflections (like all other stages) is marked by what we have called an antipathic emotional attitude—antipathic because it is the negation of its sympathetic thrust. If, in adolescence, the new sympathy arising is the potential of fidelity toward value systems to which one can relate one's identity, its antipathic counterpart is the repudiation of other such systems. Intimacy in young adulthood, naturally sympathetic, is strengthened and circumscribed by an exclusivity that disinvites outsiders, while generativity is accompanied by a rejectivity that draws strict lines against persons and groups not considered worthy of our care.

It is (almost) unnecessary to point out that all such antipathic inclinations during vast changes in history can be seemingly well rationalized in their projection on "foreign" ways of life and ideologies. These projections help to relieve the inner political or familial conditions from hostile tension and increase, say, the potential for bonding within the home boundaries.

The nuclear situation, however, exposes in an almost incomprehensible way the fact that (yes, ingenious) technology is about to eradicate (or already has) all the relative safety zones associated with the existing territorialities on earth. No matter how many children can be brought up in what territorial areas and with whose humanitarian help, only mankind as a whole can assure their survival and their future.

Something tells me that some of what we have learned to see in our time in regard to the syntonic and dystonic human potentials built into the life cycle by evolution and history are surely in need of much further study. So let me simply stress once more, take care.

REFERENCES

Erikson, E. H., with Erikson, J. M. 1948. Growth and crisis of the "healthy personality." In C. Kluckhohn and H. A. Murray, eds. *Personality in Nature, Society, and Culture*. New York: Knopf.

Lifton, R. J. 1974. In R. J. Lifton and E. Olson, eds. *Explorations in Psychohistory*. New York: Simon & Schuster.

Nichtern, S. 1983. The pursuit of the fantasy family: generational aspects. *Adolescent Psychiatry*, this volume.

3 OBSTACLES AND PATHWAYS IN THE JOURNEY FROM ADOLESCENCE TO PARENTHOOD

ALBERT J. SOLNIT

Introduction

In the second and last period of rapid growth and development of childhood, adolescents begin a search for competence in response to inner yearnings and to their community's expectations, hopes, or demands. They are reaching for physical, social, sexual, and work competence that will satisfy their need to feel unique, worthy, and capable of achieving adulthood. In this search for competence and balance, adolescents are responsive to the shaping influences and demands of their social environment at the same time as they are a vital shaping part of their environment (Solnit 1979). These counterbalancing forces, inner and outer, are often in conflict. Such conflicts constitute challenges that can become obstacles to a progressive healthy development in adolescence.

Developmental Considerations

In examining the extent of adolescents' reciprocating influence on their social and physical milieu, clinicians and developmental scholars (Blos 1979; Laufer 1975; Offer, Marohn, and Ostrov 1979; Solnit 1972, 1976) have explored adolescence as a critical phase of development, assessing the advantages and disadvantages of certain environmental and biological trends. The experiences of adolescents in our world of unrest have been complexly and significantly influenced by the rapid

14

convergence of improved health and nutritional care, when the latter is available, and the demands for more education as the institutionalized means of achieving freedom and independence.

In his crucial studies, Tanner (1971) pointed out that the average girl in the Scandinavian countries begins to menstruate at just over thirteen years of age, as opposed to seventeen years in the 1840s. In the United States, the average onset age of menarche has declined from 14.2 years in 1900 to about 12.45 today. In his reports, Tanner observed that the age at menarche had declined an average of four months per decade for the past century.

"During the last hundred years, there has been a striking tendency for children to become progressively larger at all ages [Tanner 1968]. This is known as the 'secular trend.' The magnitude of the trend in Europe and America is such that it dwarfs the differences among socioeconomic classes.

"During the same period, there has been an upward trend in adult height but to a considerably lesser degree. In earlier times the final height was not reached until twenty-five years or later, whereas now it is reached in men at eighteen or nineteen" (Tanner 1971) and often by seventeen years.

In girls the interval from the first sign of puberty to complete maturity varies from one and a half to six years. Menarche invariably occurs after peak height velocity is passed, so the tall girl can be reassured about future growth limits if her periods have begun.

In boys a similar variability occurs. The genitalia may take between two and five years to reach adult size.

As Tanner points out, the signal to start the sequence of events is given by the brain cortex, not the pituitary. Just as the brain holds the information on sex, so it holds information on maturity. Maturation is organized and stimulated. More is known about this mechanism in rats. In these animals, small amounts of sex hormones circulate from the time of birth. They inhibit the prepubertal hypothalamus from producing gonadotrophin releasers. At puberty, it is assumed, the hypothalamic cells become less sensitive to sex hormones. "The small amount of sex hormones circulating then fails to inhibit the hypothalamus and gonadotrophins are released; these stimulate the production of testosterone by the testis or estrogen by the ovary. The level of sex hormone rises until the same feedback circuit is reestablished, but now at a higher level of gonadotrophins and sex hormones. The sex hormones are now high enough to stimulate the growth

15

of secondary sex characteristics and support mating behavior'' (Tanner 1971).

Is there a relationship between earlier and greater amounts of psychosexual stimulation and earlier maturation? This is an unanswered question since the mechanism for triggering puberty in humans is still being investigated.

Tanner (1971) states, ''Some authors have supposed that the increased psychosexual stimulation consequent on modern urban living has contributed, but there is no positive evidence for this. Girls in single-sex schools have menarche at exactly the same age as girls in coeducational schools, but whether this is a fair test of difference in psychosexual stimulation is hard to say.''

We should not underestimate the effect on adolescence of our rapidly changing social environment. This includes the sexual revolution, equal rights for women, the increasing divorce rate, and the increase of single-parent families and women in the labor force. On the whole, this may lead to better options for youth. However, outside transitions that are rapid are often difficult to cope with when so much rapid change is taking place inside. Thus, our observations and theory suggest that, in adolescence, changes in the biological timetable in the direction of an earlier and more rapid maturation, and the necessity for a longer and more complicated psychosocial postponement before taking on adult responsibilities and activities, have emotional as well as social and economic implications.

The need to achieve more education and training intensifies the conflicts of the adolescent in our society. This intensification is increased and further influenced by the utilization of the newer technological capacities for perceiving and mastering our physical environment in a variety of ways. For example, instant transportation and communication offer adolescents opportunities for knowing more rapidly what is taking place in their proximal and distal environments and for greater geographic mobility. Such opportunities may enable adolescents to be able to understand and cope more effectively with their environment. At the same time, there are compelling disadvantages to what may be experienced as demands for adaptation to a rapidly changing, less stable environment. Under certain circumstances, our technological society will encourage adolescents' infantile attitudes and behavior (instant gratification and magic thinking—press a button and it happens!) more than evoking their capacity for mastery through providing acceptable, attractive channels for the expression of socially constructive and

16

satisfying behavior, that is, when increased awareness of the outer world evokes the channeling of inner resources in the service of coping and of constantly modifying, or changing, the social environment.

In order to acquire the experience and mature judgment necessary for the full liberation from childhood ties and dependency and to achieve a balance between conforming to, and actively changing, the environment according to his or her preferences, the adolescent ordinarily requires an extended education. This, in turn, leads to a prolongation of the adolescent moratorium. Such extensions may be in conflict with the increased rate of individual maturation made possible by improved nutrition and preventive health care. In fact, since there has been a consistent scarcity of jobs for youth, society has found it easiest to keep teenagers out of the labor market by inducing them to stay in school longer.

In the United States, the vast majority of teenagers are enrolled in schools. For male teenagers who leave school, the obvious option outside of a civilian job has been the military, which offers a substitute for schools as an alternative route from adolescence to adulthood. But many youths—the precise number depends on definitions, counting methodologies, and so on—remain outside the socially accepted options of school, jobs, homemaking, or the military (Levitan 1980). Ironically, the earlier and more exuberant advent of adolescent appetites, sensitivities, and creative impulses has been confronted by society's demands for more education and more specialization and by an increased rate of social change. Teenagers' sense of time is distorted by this acceleration of social and motorical changes. They feel pushed to make "big" decisions earlier than feels comfortable, given a teenager's need to dream and explore his future choices and preferences and his own volatile longings, moods, and dreams of glory as well as his fear of certain inevitabilities. An earlier, brief maturation time, in a world that demands more preparation for adult opportunities and rewards, results in an increased pressure on adolescents when they need settings that allow time for dreaming, experimenting, and exploring their choices as they prepare for adulthood.

In a report[1] of a Conference on Adolescent Behavior and Health (1978) organized by the Institute of Medicine, it was stated: "Early adolescents are attentive and responsive to the social environment, especially those aspects that reflect the youth culture. This heightened awareness of the social milieu is coupled with involvement in the rapidly changing physiological effects of puberty. These changes predispose to a preoccupation with body image. For many there are concerns about factors influencing health, growth, and development. Feelings of isolation, purposelessness, and boredom may become manifest during early adolescence. If not countered or constructively allayed, they can lead to maladaptive and health-damaging behavior!"

Detours

Adolescents' susceptibility to, and interest in, substance abuse, especially alcohol and marijuana (mood changers), and their interest in the invitation to participate in, and to become organized by, exotic or mystical cults, can be understood as high-risk environmental influences or as experiences sought by adolescents expressing unresolved conflicts and needs through symptomatic behavior. It is clarifying to view this process as two questions:

1. Which adolescents actively seek out such opportunities?

2. Assuming the undesirability of experiences with alcohol and other drugs, or the influence of autonomy-depriving cults on young men and women who voluntarily submit to such experiences and programs, how does the adolescent's active seeking of such experiences provide a better understanding of his problems?

The adolescent's need to be active in his own search for relief and mastery also suggests the need for competitive options that are more promising in terms of resolving these developmental and psychiatric disturbances of adolescence rather than of complicating them. How do we as a society create, support, or discourage the alternatives that promote healthy or unhealthy behavior?

In the examination of the adolescent's search for competence, it is useful in mapping out this developmental terrain to examine four developmental tasks (Blos 1979). They are:

1. The loosening of childhood ties to parents and the new self-definition–individuation that proceeds to the crystallization of the adult personality.

2. The reworking and reintegration of the residues of past unsolved conflicts, deprivations, and trauma.

3. The establishment and clarification of the sense of oneself as having a unique history, a continuity from child to adult with the gradual intellectual and emotional awareness of the inevitability of life, death, and limitations of function. This developmental ac-

quisition is also associated normatively with the capacity to tolerate a certain amount of depression.

4. The resolution of sexual identity in which the adolescent moves from intuitive to explicit choices in the integration of biological sexuality with the adult sex role.

Another central task of adolescence is the elaboration and refinement of the capacity to differentiate between external objective reality and inner subjective reality. While the maturational process provides an increased capacity for adaptation and reality testing, nevertheless there are also the accompanying normative regressive forces characteristic of adolescence. These regressive reactions are observed in the unevenness and eruptibility of moods and drive energies. These include being in, and out of, synchrony with other ego capacities, including self-esteem, as well as advancing intellectual acquisitions and those progressive and regressive intellectual, sexual, and emotional capacities that are interwoven in identity formation. Thus, at the same time that there is an increased capacity to recognize and cope with reality, there is also an intensification of self-preoccupation. These alternating, and sometimes simultaneous, demands recurrently interfere with the struggle to discern and respond effectively at the same time to the external objective reality and the inner subjective demands.

It is an essential characteristic of human development, especially vivid in the adolescent period, that regressive experiences are prerequisites for mobilizing the mental resources in preparation for forward steps in development. When the balance is delicate and unstable, as is normative in contemporary adolescence, it is the response of the social environment—the invitations that promote the dynamic balance of progressive and regressive developmental forces—that reflects the cultural preferences and patterns of a given society and period of history.

In recent years there has been a challenge to the view that normatively adolescence is a period of psychological turmoil and instability. The smooth, relatively steady, and agreeable surface behavior of many adolescents has been interpreted by some experts as evidence that "adolescents, as a whole, are not in turmoil, not deeply disturbed, not at the mercy of their impulses, not resistant to parental values, not politically active or rebellious" (Adelson 1979, p. 37).

Psychoanalytic insight, in need of periodic rediscovery, has demonstrated that surface behavior of adolescence and data emerging from nonclinical interviews and questionnaires do not yield an accurate reflection of the inner instability, disharmony, and turmoil that characterize normative adolescence.

Each view is a useful one, if the limits of these formulations are kept in mind. To know that a teenager is behaviorally doing well in academic, athletic, and social activities, as viewed from the outside, does not correlate and should not be expected to correlate with the inner mental and emotional experiences of that same young man or woman. The moods, fantasies, dreams, secret fears, and wishes, that is, the painful conflicts of normative adolescence, are detectable in psychoanalytic treatment or in other settings in which subjective experiences and longings are ego syntonic, even though they are not observable in research efforts based on one or two nonclinical interviews and group observations or questionnaire data. Each of these approaches is valid within the limitations of the particular method used and of the theoretical assumptions involved. In comparing these two views of the adolescent experience, surface behavior, and inner private experiences, I am reminded of the metaphor that adolescents have two special mirrors that characterize their behavior and experience. When one sees the adolescent reflected in one mirror, his body and behavior are sharply focused, enlarged, and accelerated according to the rate of growth and according to the expectation and vision of the observer. When one sees the adolescent in the mirror of his inner subjective experience, the reflection is one in which definition, color, sensuousness, heat, and depth of perspective are changing in their intensity, in their relationship to the images reflected in the first mirror of body surface and behavior and to the tolerance and expectation of the observer. Clinicians should also think of adolescents with their two mirrors as providing beautiful, at times painful, reflections of our social environment.

Each adolescent comes to terms with the unfinished business of his childhood as a preparation for the wider social stage of adulthood. For example, the treatment of disturbed adolescents and observations of well-functioning teenagers indicate that their wishes to remain close to parents and the conflicting urge to become independent of them are a regular feature of adolescent development. The behavioral and psychological manifestation of this characteristic conflict and its resolution is variable and can appear in many direct or disguised forms. Repeatedly, we have observed that the fit between the individual adolescent's search for balanced competence and the social supports for, or the obstacles to, acquiring and expressing competence is crucial. This fit reflects the characteristic reactions of each family or culture in terms of facilitating or discouraging competence in adolescence. To the degree that familial and cultural opportunities favor facilitation, the teenager is able to move smoothly toward a more mature relationship with parents. This transition leads to increasing independence, without the need for emphasizing or distorting the normative assertiveness and rebelliousness of adolescence.

In early adolescence, during transient periods of subjective instability, of feeling out of control or not feeling certain that one has control, the search for competence becomes a powerful yearning. At these times the teenager, striving for something that will give hope and satisfaction, seeks to reduce and channel the internal volcanic eruptions of feelings and longings in order to cope with the turbulence that may characterize the inner experience of adolescence. It is well to keep in mind that the adolescent is simultaneously pulled by regressive forces and pushed by maturational thrusts. As a result, almost all of the adolescent's felt needs are psychologically conflicted in the following ways:

1. The need to relinquish ties with parents, the primary love objects, is painfully opposed by the regressive attraction exerted by the revival of childhood yearnings.

2. The need to find and become himself as an increasingly independent person is complicated by his real dependence on the persons against whom he has to rebel and on his old "crowd" of friends and peers, who commonly drift apart as time goes on.

3. An interest in, and need for, lofty, respectable ideals and values that are his own are, to a considerable extent, fueled by (less lofty) sexual and aggressive appetitive impulses and longings.

4. The need to reintegrate or reorganize various components of the personality structure may require more time than the tensions created by such a restructuring permit, frequently leading the adolescent to adopt a restricted or premature solution in order to gain relief from the intolerable tensions of inner conflict and outer social demands or expectations.

Such developmental conflicts, tugs, and pulls often do not appear as overt or observable behavior.

Utilizing clinical psychoanalytic observations of adolescent boys and girls, ages fourteen to eighteen, as well as direct observations of this age group in different settings, I have found it becomes increasingly useful to assume that the search for physical, social, sexual, and intellectual competence[2] represents a primary developmental task of mid adolescence. The degree to which this task (or need) is mastered or not can be a useful guide in evaluating and understanding healthy as well as deviant development in adolescence. For parents, educators, and employers, this assumption of the adolescent search for competence can be used as a guide in planning for work as well as for educational and social opportunities for youth. This view of the adolescent's search for competence can also be useful to adults who wish to work toward understanding and improving the constructive influence of a community's standards for acceptable behavior in adolescence.

Discussion

The adolescent's search for competence is an adaptive and defensive reaction to the unsettling of the school-aged child's self-esteem and confidence in social and cognitive skills associated with the rapid pubertal unfolding of maturational and developmental capacities. These proceed rapidly, usually in dysynchrony or disharmony with each other. Along with rapid emotional and intellectual changes, there is an acceleration of physical growth, a characteristic of the first phase of postpubertal changes. This evidence of physical health, desirable in itself, may complicate the psychological task because the relatively rapid sensory and motor changes, alteration of body contour and the body image, are also a part of the changing personality.

Two metaphors illuminate this developmental perspective.

One metaphor is of a race in which all the competitors start together, and the goal is to have them finish at about the same time. However, in the course of adolescence, first the impulsive side of the personality, the volcanic drives, is ahead, then the ego forges ahead, then the conscience and moral side of the personality, the superego, becomes dominant—not always in a kindly way. These powerful intellectual, psychological, and emotional forces, which formerly were in relative harmony in the latency child, vie with each other as life's experiences, education, and the commitment of parents, siblings, and grandparents ideally enable the "racers" within to become parts of a single integrated person in which the parts become subservient to the synthesis of a clear, attractive, unique identity. Thus, the healthy adolescent's search for competence facilitates the unfolding of a unique personality, prepared to feel the zest and tolerate the depressive aspects of a full life of love and work. Parents often feel jarred by the "race," forgetting that what had been invested in care and model-setting patterns will emerge in the "new" adult who is establishing himself. Under such provocation, parents often lose the desirable balance of admiration for, and resentment of, these demanding, challenging, rebelling young men and women.

We cherish our representatives for the future, a bid for immortality, when they perform as we wish. We resent our replacements who require us to share our limited resources with them as they remind us of our own adolescence.

The second metaphor concentrates on the adolescent experience itself. "But when, by what test, by what indication does manhood [or womanhood] commence? Physically, by one criterion [and a changing one at that]; legally by another; morally by a third; intellectually by a fourth—and all indefinite. Equator, absolute equator, there is none," as Thomas DeQuincy said over a century ago (Kiell 1964).

In a recently published report by the United States Committee for the Study of National Service (1979), a panel of distinguished American leaders gives voice to the need for a national policy that responds to youth's search for competence in a rapidly changing society. The report gives balanced attention to three principles on which they base their recommendations: (1) in the interest of the social and psychological development of young people, including the considerations of an enhanced sense of altruism for the common good and a more positive self-esteem that is associated with work that develops competence and the capacity to feel realistically responsible for others; (2) in the interest of viewing young people as a national resource that is useful and cherished; and (3) in the interest of enabling youth to join together in ameliorating social disturbance, distress, and deprivation in the community. The panel and its study director, Roger Landrum, call attention to James's (1910) *The Moral Equivalent of War* as a means for ". . . gaining a generation with a new sense of 'civic discipline' outside the context of war." This argument is elaborated and refined in Coleman (1972).

Others question the recommendations inherent in these three principles or assumptions. The reservations are articulated in the following statement (Levitan 1980):

In a society where pluralism is dominant, the case for a voluntary national service sponsored by the federal government is far from clear. The United States abounds with voluntary organizations doing good works: churches, fraternal organizations and a multitude of other groups helping advance worthy causes. In line with past practices and still widely held values, good works should best be left to individuals, private organizations, and indeed, youth as well as adults, each to serve the nation, their communities, and their neighbors in different ways. This can best be achieved by encouraging youth to exercise their available options. A youth with a potential for playing the fiddle and becoming a concert violinist could best serve by enrolling in a conservatory. A youth who is 6'8", and still growing, might make the greatest contribution by playing college basketball for the greater glory of his alma mater and by preparing to maximize the Gross National Product. Others can best serve by acting as missionaries for their churches. The bulk of youngsters can best serve their country and themselves by learning a trade or enrolling in college to learn a bit of Shakespeare and study the mysteries of integral calculus.

In brief, there is no question that the United States has experienced a job deficit for youth. Society has made various efforts to provide for a growing number of socially useful activities which employ teenagers. A strong case can be made for expanding the number of jobs available.

Underlying these studies and recommendations is the determination of respected social scientists, educators, and national leaders to respond constructively to the developmental needs and capabilities of our youth as expressed in the search for competence. These reports recognize the fit between this developmental search and our national effort to achieve social policies that simultaneously lead to meeting human developmental needs and advancing the common good in a democratic society.

Conclusion

It is not until the healthy or normal completion of adolescent developmental tasks that the individual has confidence in his sense of self and in the his sense of who can be important to him in an abiding way. With a favorable balance of development, the search for competence

ALBERT J. SOLNIT

can culminate during adulthood in an "original" orchestration of those intellectual and emotional forces that characterize a particular and unique person. This orchestration also is apparent as the adult feels physically, sexually, socially, and intellectually competent. Such a synthesis is reflected in the mature choices of loved persons and careers that have the stability, predictability, and consonance of healthy adulthood. In the best sense of the word "unique," each adolescent strives for a unique future, one that is a constructive continuation of a unique past.

NOTES

1. Workshop on Family and Social Environment, June 26 and 27, 1978. Cochaired by Beatrix Hamburg, M.D., and Albert J. Solnit, M.D., at Conference on Adolescent Behavior and Health, Division of Health Sciences Policy, Division of Health Promotion and Disease Prevention, Institute of Medicine, National Academy of Sciences, Washington, D.C., October.

2. Adequacy is defined as "possession of a required skill, knowledge, qualification or capacity"; *Random House Dictionary of the English Language* (unabridged ed. [New York: Random House, 1966]). Competent is defined as "well qualified, capable, fit, sufficient, adequate"; *Webster's New World Dictionary of the American Language* (college ed. [New York: World, 1966]).

REFERENCES

Adelson, J. 1979. Adolescence and the generalization gap. *Psychology Today,* February.

Blos, P. 1979. *The Adolescent Passage.* New York: International Universities Press.

Coleman, J. S. 1972. *Youth: Transition to Adulthood.* Chicago: University of Chicago Press.

Committee for the Study of National Service. 1979. *Youth and the Needs of the Nation.* Washington, D.C.: Potomac Institute, January.

James, W. 1910. *The Moral Equivalent of War.* International Conciliation, no. 27. New York: Carnegie Endowment for International Peace.

Kiell, N. 1964. *The Universal Experience of Adolescence.* New York: International Universities Press.

Laufer, M. 1975. *Adolescent Disturbance and Breakdown.* Harmondsworth: Penguin.

Levitan, S. 1980. What shall we do for (or to) our youth in the 1980s? *New Generation* 60(2, 3): 7–12.

Offer, D.; Marohn, R.; and Ostrov, E. 1979. *The Psychological World of the Juvenile Delinquent.* New York: Basic.

Petersen, A. 1979. Can puberty come any earlier? *Psychology Today,* February.

Solnit, A. J. 1972. Adolescence and the changing reality. In I. M. Marcus, ed. *Currents in Psychoanalysis.* New York: International Universities Press.

Solnit, A. J. 1976. Inner and outer changes in adolescence. *Journal of the Philadelphia Association for Psychoanalysis* 3(3): 43–46.

Solnit, A. J. 1979. The adolescent's search for competence. *Children Today* 8(6): 13–15.

Tanner, J. M. 1968. Earlier maturation in man. *Scientific American* 218:20–27.

Tanner, J. M. 1971. Sequence tempo and individual variation in the growth and development of boys and girls aged 12 to 16. *Daedalus* 100:907–930.

4 THE PURSUIT OF THE FANTASY FAMILY: GENERATIONAL ASPECTS

SOL NICHTERN

The traditional concept of the family is that of a group of persons related by blood: parents, children, uncles, aunts, and cousins identified as coming from a common progenitor. Family relationships are biologic in origin and result in a defined set of characteristics; there can be only one mother and one father to a family. These biologic parents are the most significant in the life of children by definition; other combinations of parents and children defy this finite system and become surrogates, aberrations, myths, or fantasies.

Major changes, however, seem to be occurring within family units challenging this traditional concept. The Census Bureau (Hacker 1982) reports that, from 1970 to 1980, the total number of households increased 24.8 percent, while the general population increased only 11.5 percent. The number of persons in the average household declined from 3.14 to 2.75 during this same period. The number of families with unmarried heads grew by 52.3 percent. By 1980, 23.4 percent of all children age seventeen years or under were not living with both biologic parents. This was true of 57.8 percent of black children and 17.3 percent of white children. Nonfamily households grew 73.5 percent to a total of more than twenty million. This increase resulted from young people marrying later or preferring to live alone while single, along with a marked increase in divorced persons. It is particularly significant that the period from 1970 to 1980 saw the creation of more than fifteen million new households of which 55.6 percent were of the nonfamily variety. Of the remaining 44.4 percent, the majority were those with a single-head family. Only 22 percent of the total household growth of this decade came from couples who were married and in the position to uphold the traditional concept of family and family household. Therefore, the definition of family as a group of persons related by blood or marriage may no longer be adequate for an understanding of the nature of family relationships.

Recurrent themes among the thoughts and behavior patterns of adolescents reveal their search for special relationships or households of their own choice and making. The origin of this search can be traced to inner conflicts rooted in the reappearance during adolescence of problems associated with individuation and separation needs. Who they are (psychological self) and what they are (sexual self) must be redefined within a continuing struggle for maturity. Most conflicts are accompanied by some impairment of impulse control, confusion of ideas, breakdown of values, and distortion of feelings. These characteristics blend with the nature of conflicts within the turmoil of adolescence, creating new symbolic constructs.

A fantasy family is one such construct. Fantasy families provide the adolescent with the means of reconstituting and preserving the self: impulses can be controlled with a clearly defined set of rules of conduct; confusion of ideas can be curbed or eliminated with simplified or overdetermined relationships; values can be constructed and accepted without question; and feelings can be redefined as needed. This system provides a structure for existing with the conflicts until they are resolved and serves as the vehicle for the transmission of family values. When the conflicts are not readily resolved, a new, often different, and persistent symbolic construct of family is established, reflecting the turmoil of adolescence rather than the biologic family of origin. This makes the fantasy family of adolescence significant to generativity (Erikson 1968) and establishes psychological origins for the concepts of family equal to, and sometimes more important than, its biologic origin.

The most common fantasy family of adolescence bears a marked similarity to the family experienced within early childhood, permitting traditional and parental values to be preserved and transmitted from one generation to the next. This fantasy family construct is similar to that of early childhood because of the reappearance of the same individuation and separation problems and reflects the same patterns of resolution of childhood conflicts. There is little room for the persistence of unresolved conflict where family values and relationships are strong and clearly determined. Controls, ideas, values, and feelings are established quickly and used effectively for the resolution of conflict.

The fantasy family of adolescence cannot exist or survive under some circumstances. Families within agriculturally based societies are determined by culture and economy to be similar. The available family constructs are consistently the same, as are the rules of conduct, the concepts of relationships, and the values and feelings of one to another. Adolescence, as a differentiating stage of transition, is less significant. Children become adults within their family with little need for change. Alternatives are few. Often, the adolescent is provided with rites of passage to adult role and responsibility. These rites of passage are, themselves, significant symbolic constructs eliminating the need for other fantasies. Now, the preserved rituals of some of these ancient rites of passage as well as social practices of contemporary industrial societies generate anxiety and conflict within many adolescents. They no longer appear to be serving their original purpose and yet continue to have so much of past symbolic meaning that they may activate and fuel unresolved conflicts of childhood.

Certain types of fantasy families are associated with the reappearance of unresolved individuation and separation problems of childhood during adolescence. Some of the intense attachments of the earlier developmental period may be preserved and remain quiescent until the turmoil of adolescence causes them to reappear. These attachments are strong enough to determine many of the relationships sought by the adolescent while providing the structure for a family prototype. Thus, the adolescent boy may be attracted to the girl "just like the girl who married dear old Dad" and behave just like the boy that dear old Mom really wanted. The pursuit of these relationships becomes finalized in the oppositional stance of one generation to another.

The opposite may occur as well. Adolescence may bring a strong incestuous component to persistent early attachments, making these family relationships unacceptable as a model. The adolescent must move toward other kinds of relationships and family constructs in order to prevent this. A common resolution of this conflictual state is the recruitment of adolescent relationships and peer grouping for the family model. The resulting family construct becomes overly determined by the rules governing peer interactions within adolescence.

An example of the fantasy family with a total break from its generational predecessor can be seen within our drug culture. Drug use by adolescents appears to be akin to a modern rite of passage. Its initial use seems to correlate with the onset of adolescence. Its continuing use appears to correlate with interactions among adolescents. Its persistent use seems to be related to the lack of resolution of adolescent conflicts leading to the recruitment of the fantasy of being part of a family group made up of peers. Order is achieved and relationships are determined through the procurement, distribution, and use of drugs. A study of the children of drug users (Nichtern 1973a) indicated that the drug-addicted parents' only linkage to each other appeared to be their use of drugs. Also, many of the drug-addicted mothers were unwilling to consider surrender of parental rights, even after they had totally abandoned their children. Their unwillingness was accompanied by repeated expressions of the desire to reconstitute a family—though none had ever existed, and their child had been born out of wedlock with an uncertain paternity. These expressions took place in the face of abandonment of mother and infant by the father of the child, extensive social disorder, continuing involvement with drug usage, and long periods of absence from their children. None of these facts made any difference to their ambition to offer their children a complete and intact family life. Here, pursuit of the fantasy of family becomes finalized in substitution of the construct of grouping for family.

Part of this same process has extended into the management and treatment of the drug abuser. Many treatment programs for the drug abuser are based on family-like groupings. Some who have given up the use of drugs become drug counselors, with the equivalent surrogate parental rights over those who are still drug abusers. The members of the group remain together within the drug treatment program, and loyalty to the group and its objectives is essential. An unusual experience associated with some of these programs has been the exclusion of non–drug users as being alien and unable to understand fully or cope with the problems of drug use. One effort to intervene in behalf of the children of drug abusers was totally frustrated by the staff of a drug-abuse program because they did not want "outsiders" involved with the members of their group. They claimed that only they could address themselves to the real problems of the offspring of the drug abuser.

The inability to accept multiple relationships may be another consequence of persistent early attachments and result in yet another type of fantasy family. Only the attachment of the resulting symbiosis remains significant. There is no family construct possible beyond the symbiotic relationship. The consequence is the destruction of the generational family. Any intruder to the symbiotic relationship must be excluded. This leads to the breakdown of existing family ties, to divorce, to disruption of peer relations, and to a fantasy family composed only of the symbiotic partners coming from two separate generations. Each of the generational partners views himself or herself as complete and self-sufficient. They usually live in intimacy and harmony until the symbiosis is threatened or until pubescence heralds the introduction of adolescence to the younger member of the alliance. The binding nature of the symbiotic relationship and the unacceptability of peers for significant relationships intensifies the conflicts of adolescence to an unbearable degree. The only resolution of such conflicts is regression by the adolescent partner to a very dependent existence. The earliest construct of family that satisfied the original needs of the symbiotic relationship is sought. If this type of dependency is tolerable, it goes right on serving as the family construct. If it is not tolerable, it leads to a breakdown of the symbiotic system or of one or both of the individuals involved in the symbiotic relationship. Adolescents caught up in such intense turmoil can be identified as seriously disturbed individuals. They lend themselves to ready recruitment by any individual offering them the opportunity for a dependent, substitute, symbiotic relationship within the construct of such a primitive fantasy family. The Manson family may have been this kind of fantasy family, serving the intense needs of disrupted symbiotic relationships.

There are a number of special areas of human interaction affected by the construct of the fantasy family. Among them are child abuse, adoption, and foster care. Neglected and abused children often grow up to become abusing parents. Follow-up studies (Polansky, Hally, and Polansky 1975; Polansky, Chalmers, Buttenweiser, and Williams 1981) of abused children revealed them as more likely to become delinquent and more likely to be involved in violence against people than other delinquents. Another study (Young 1964) of parents implicated in neglect revealed a significant incidence of drug usage, including alcohol, as well as mental illness and a larger than usual number of children per family. Many of the parents appeared childlike, exhibiting dependence, impulsivity, inability to carry responsibility, poor judgment, narcissistic orientation, and other evidences of failure to mature.

Understanding the continuing investment in children by adults who have themselves been the product of neglect and abuse should include awareness of the construct of the fantasy family. As these individuals

31

reached adolescence, conflicts about the abuse they received as children stimulated the fantasy of being part of a good family. Once this fantasy became entrenched, the ideal was pursued within their fantasy, while their own abuse determined their behavior. They may become recruited as producers of children (often many) through acts of impulse and abusers of children by the perpetuation of their conflicts. They have little awareness of their participation in the abuse and neglect of their children. They are capable of rationalizing the disorder of their family by illogical judgments. They seem to have difficulty in applying acceptable values and standards. Many of the firstborn of such neglecting families are conceived out of wedlock and during the parents' adolescence. Not only are the children the product of acting out but the families into which they are born remain the vehicles for continuous acting out by all who are part of them—child or adult. Thus the generational link for abuse becomes established and transmitted by way of the fantasy family.

Adoption provides fertile soil for the construct of the fantasy family. Adopted individuals may have impressions about their biologic roots distorted by the adoptive process. Vague and confused information concerning circumstances and reasons for relinquishing parental rights is common, and, even when the information is accurate, expected conflicts surrounding individuation and separation activate fantasies and distortions. This leads the efforts to resolve the conflicts of adolescence, concerning identity, with adoption more influenced by imagination. When nothing is known about the biologic parents, they can become a total product of imagination and used as needed within the construct of the fantasy family. Content and use become unrelated and subject to distortion. When the biologic parents are known, reasons for giving their child for adoption become part of a process for justifying the sense of abandonment associated with any individuation and separation problems. At the same time, the many reasons for adults' adopting children are often obscured. These reasons frequently involve the special needs of the adopting adults and, more often than not, are invested in problems of identity. Infertility, inadequacy, unresolved conflicts, and other reasons prompt adults to adopt but also stimulate the recruitment of the construct of their fantasy families that strongly affects child-rearing practices and parent-child interactions. The consequences are many and unpredictable. In some instances, the adoptee, during adolescence, denies the significance of family, biologic or adoptive, in order to cope with the confusion of his or her own and parents' fantasies. In other instances, they may choose one or the other reason as significant and incorporate their choice into their fantasy family, permitting their selection to overdetermine their thoughts and behavior. The search for ''the real family'' by the adoptee almost always begins during adolescence and may continue throughout the life span of the adoptee, unrelated to success or failure within the search. It is, however, finally determined that it is their own identity they are seeking.

The complexities of foster care are so great (Nichtern 1973b) that the fantasy of family dominates everyone within the system—the children who come for care, the parents who bring their children for care, the foster parents who provide the care, and the adults who run the system. Foster children are plagued by the confusion of too many parents—biologic, foster, and professionals—and too many families—their own, foster families, and institutional settings with their surrogate families. These circumstances lead to an easy breakdown of boundaries within the child of images of self and family. Most foster children have no place to escape the confusion except into fantasy. They construct a fantasy family that meets their own inner needs while responding to their realities of foster placement. The consequence of this process is to see every possible combination of family construct within the fantasy: orphans become preoccupied with their biological families; siblings assume parental roles to other siblings; unusual and intense attachments develop between children and surrogate parents; bondings develop between children and adults that reflect internal need more than correctness or adequacy of choice; natural parents may be rejected while inadequate surrogate parents are accepted; and, in too many instances, only the fantasy family becomes important to the foster child, so that no real human attachments develop, and the child is damaged to the point of not being able to have meaningful relations with others.

The nature of foster care recruits all who come to it to contribute to the fantasy of family. The system of foster care is built on the assumption that a surrogate parent can be found to provide the essentials of nurturing care and on the myth that a system can be developed to give a child a nurturing family. Indeed, we can find surrogate parents and families for most of our children when the need arises, but we cannot assure them the quality of the nurturing or ignore the inner need of the children to define some of their own parameters of care and family. These parameters are derived from their own individuation and separation needs. An awareness and response to these needs would permit us to help the children to a better balance between their fantasy and reality. This balance might help them achieve a cohesive identity and the nurturing relationships necessary for healthy development.

Conclusions

The recognition of the existence of a fantasy family permits a more appropriate response to the needs of individuals. However, the recognition of its special characteristics provides us with a system by which we can account for the transmission of values from one generation to another while also explaining the manner in which the transmitted values can be altered. The transmission may even reflect the changes within society as expressed by the individuals' response to their adolescent turmoil.

REFERENCES

Alfaro, H. D. 1978. Summary report on the relationship between child abuse and neglect and larger socially deviant behavior. New York: New York State Assembly Select Committee on Child Abuse.

Erikson, E. H. 1968. *Identity, Youth and Crisis*. New York: Norton.

Hacker, A. 1982. Farewell to the family. *New York Review of Books*. March 18.

Nichtern, S. 1973a. The children of drug users. *Journal of the American Academy of Child Psychiatry* 12:24–31.

Nichtern, S. 1973b. The care of dependent children. *Journal of the American Academy of Child Psychiatry* 12:393–399.

Polansky, N. A.; Chalmers, M. A.; Buttenweiser, E.; and Williams, D. P. 1981. *Damaged Parents*. Chicago: University of Chicago Press.

Polansky, N. A.; Hally, C.; and Polansky, N. F. 1975. *Profile of Neglect*. Washington, D.C.: Public Service Administration Department of HEW.

Young, L. 1964. *Wednesday's Children: A Study of Child Neglect and Abuse*. New York: McGraw-Hill.

5 THE ACADEMIA, THE PSEUDO-COMMUNITY, AND THE ARMY IN THE DEVELOPMENT OF IDENTITY

DAVID A. ROTHSTEIN

As therapists we ask what a symptom does *for* a person as well as what it does *to* the person. Only if we begin to understand why a patient needs his or her illness, what function it is serving for the patient, can we begin to help the patient meet that need and fulfill that function in a more adaptive way.

This chapter was prepared for a panel at the May 1982 ASAP annual meeting. The title of the panel, "Violent Solutions to the Identity Crisis," implicitly recognizes the above principle. It implies that the ordinarily undesirable phenomenon of violence can perform a function: it can be a *solution*. Further, it suggests what one such function can be: a solution to the identity crisis.

In previous studies of violent behavior in individuals, particularly presidential assassins, potential assassins, and threateners (Rothstein 1964, 1965a, 1965b, 1966, 1968a, 1968b, 1971a, 1971b, 1971c, 1973, 1975), I had found that identity problems were among those factors that led to the violent (or potentially violent) behavior. The title for the panel stimulated the further insight that, if problems with identity led to violent behavior, it might be that the violent behavior provided, or at least promised to provide, some form of a solution for those problems. I therefore decided to investigate whether this might be the case. Is it true that people can and do use violence to solve their identity crises? And, if so, how does violence contribute to identity formation?

I propose to suggest and, I hope, to demonstrate here: that violence can play a part in solutions to the identity crisis, not only for those disturbed individuals who become the outcasts of society as patients or prisoners but also for those who make up the fabric of society; that violence plays a part in larger-scale group and national identity; and that there is an interplay between the violent solutions on an individual level and those on a larger-scale social level. The violence inherent in the socially approved solutions may foster the violence of certain disturbed individuals. More often, it "goes underground" in the solutions of the greater majority of the relatively "well-adjusted" individuals, but the solutions found by these individuals contribute to the eventual resurfacing of the violence on the larger-scale social level, in particular in the form of war. War is not necessarily a part of basic human nature. It is a social institution perpetuated by social phenomena that interact with individual psychology, particularly in the crucial area of adolescent identity formation.

Case Studies

CASE 1: RON

Ron wrote about the pleasures and pains of adolescence and about his ideals, ambitions, and dreams.

He recalled the pleasures in his bodily sensations and the joy of mastering his athletic abilities. He remembered his parents proudly watching as he and his brother worked out on the parallel bars which his father had built in the backyard.

Although he was shy, Ron was also able to recognize his exhibitionistic feelings. He wanted to be a hero, to be stared at and talked about in the hallways. He had an idea of what it was to be a hero:

> Every Saturday afternoon we'd go down to the movies in the shopping center and watch gigantic prehistoric birds breathe fire, and war movies with John Wayne and Audie Murphy. . . . I'll never forget Audie Murphy in *To Hell and Back*. At the end he jumps on top of a flaming tank that's just about to explode and grabs the machine gun blasting it into the German lines. He was so brave I had chills running up and down my back, wishing it were me up there. . . . Castiglia and I saw *The Sands of Iwo Jima* together. . . . They showed the men raising the flag on Iwo Jima with the marines' hymn still playing. . . . Like Mickey Mantle and

36

the fabulous New York Yankees, John Wayne . . . became one of my heroes.

But Ron and his friends were not mere passive observers:

We'd go home and make up movies like the ones we'd just seen or the ones that were on TV night after night. We'd use our Christmas toys—the Matty Mattel machine guns and grenades, the little green plastic soldiers. . . . On Saturdays after the movies all the guys would go down to Sally's Woods. . . . We turned the woods into a battlefield. We set ambushes, then led gallant attacks. . . . Then we'd walk out of the woods like the heroes we knew we would become when we were men.

They also made plans and formed a bond:

We studied the Marine Corps Guidebook and Richie brought over some beautiful pamphlets with very sharp-looking marines on the covers. We read them in my basement for hours and just as we dreamed of playing for the Yankees someday, we dreamed of becoming United States Marines and fighting our first war and we made a solemn promise that year that the day we turned seventeen we were both going down to the marine recruiter at the shopping center in Levittown and sign up for the United States Marine Corps.

Ron looked up to his father and remembered his relationship to him in positive terms. He described how proud he had felt to help his father with tasks such as repairs around the house. Nevertheless, Ron did not wish to identify completely with his father, who worked as a checker in a supermarket:

I didn't want to be like my Dad, coming home from the A&P every night. He was a strong man, a good man, but it made him so tired, it took all the energy out of him. I didn't want to be like that, working in that stinking A&P, six days a week, twelve hours a day. I wanted to be somebody. I wanted to make something out of my life.

The marines provided a powerful ideal for Ron—and a way to reach that ideal. He was enthralled when marine recruiters came to speak to his senior class. "It was like all the movies and all the books and all the dreams of becoming a hero come true" (Kovic 1976).

So Ron joined the marines.

Of course, in reading his book, one already knows that Ron Kovic has been wounded in Vietnam and has become a paraplegic.

CASE 2: DR. S.

Dr. S. remembered a private society of his adolescence. At age fourteen, he and five friends formed a literary and philosophical society which met on Saturday afternoons to discuss philosophical, scientific, and aesthetic matters:

> Periodically, we may have reenacted literary or historical fantasies. . . . It was then that I began my reading of Freud and continued to cherish the wish that, impossible as it seemed, I might one day become an analyst.

Dr. S. recalled that his real determination to become an analyst and follow Freud originated even before adolescence, when he was eleven. His father had suffered a business failure, and his mother had become quite depressed as a result. This resulted in considerable disillusionment with his parents. Not long afterward, he was fascinated by a movie about a good twin and a bad twin who could be distinguished only by psychological investigation. "I soon learned about psychoanalysis, and I was led to a serious pursuit of my career."

He also described an intense relationship which he had with an older boy during the ages of eleven to fourteen, before he had formed the literary and philosophical society:

> We confided in one another and shared curiosity and interest in sexual matters. We also engaged in various fantasy projects. We frequently pretended we were boy detectives, the heroes of an adventure story. Several times we followed people, sometimes across the city, with the hope that we would learn something secret and special. A little more persistently, we conceived of a newspaper and even produced one copy after having sold several subscriptions to neighbors. [Wolf, Gedo, and Terman 1972]

CASE 3: WINSTON

Winston began school at age seven:

> How I hated this school, and what a life of anxiety I lived there for more than two years. . . . I counted the days and the hours to the end of every term, when I should return home from this hateful servitude and range my soldiers in line of battle on the nursery floor. [Churchill 1930]

At age thirteen he entered Harrow. Academically, he was placed in the bottom form of the school. He discovered that he could rise above his lowly position by learning 1,200 lines of Macaulay for a prize. For the rest of his life he was able to recite these lines with gusto and relish. His son noted in later years that these verses evoked a stirring patriotism which abided with Winston forever and was the mainspring of his political conduct. His youthful patriotism was also stirred by the Harrow school songs. Later, during World War II, attending an annual singing of these school songs, he said with lively emotion, "Listening to those boys singing all those well-remembered songs I could see myself 50 years before singing with them those tales of great deeds and of great men and wondering with intensity how I could ever do something glorious for my country" (Churchill 1966).

He took great interest in the school rifle corps, which he joined almost immediately, and took part in his first field day, which took the form of a battle. He found the battle very exciting. He wrote to his mother about the experience and included a map of the positions.

Winston was disappointed that for eighteen months his father did not come to Harrow to see what his school life was like. During the term when Winston was fourteen, his father expressed the desire that Winston go into the army. His father had been much impressed by the obvious enthusiasm with which Winston was describing his outings with the rifle corps, but Winston attributed the decision to another reason (Churchill 1930):

> I was now embarked on a military career. This orientation was entirely due to my collection of Soldiers. I had ultimately nearly fifteen hundred. They were all of one size, all British, and organized as an infantry division with a cavalry brigade. My brother Jack commanded the hostile army. . . .

The day came when my father himself paid a formal visit of inspection. All the troops were arranged in the correct formation of attack. He spent twenty minutes studying the scene—which was really impressive—At the end he asked me if I would like to go into the Army. I thought it would be splendid to command an Army, so I said "Yes" at once: and immediately I was taken at my word. For years I thought my father with his experience and flair had discerned in me the qualities of military genius. But I was told later that he had only come to the conclusion that I was not clever enough to go to the Bar. However that may be, the toy soldiers turned the current of my life. Henceforward, all my education was directed to passing into Sandhurst [the Royal Military College] and afterwards to the technical details of the profession of arms.

Accordingly, Winston joined the army class shortly before he was fifteen. When he was sixteen, Winston built a "den" at the family's new country house. This was a hut constructed of mud and planks and carpeted with straw inside. With his brother Jack, his cousins, and other children on the estate, Winston built intricate fortifications around it, including a moat and a drawbridge. A large homemade elastic catapult which propelled green apples guarded the entrance. "Winston now graduated from drilling his toy soldiers . . . to drilling his brother, his cousins and his other 'volunteers' . . ." (Churchill 1966).

Winston was deeply interested in his work at Sandhurst. His father had his bookseller send Winston books on warfare, including "a number of histories dealing with the American Civil, Franco-German and Russo-Turkish Wars, which were then our latest and best specimens of wars."

Sometimes he was invited to dine at the Staff College (Churchill 1930):

Here the study was of divisions, Army Corps and even whole armies; of bases, of supplies, and lines of communication and railway strategy. This was thrilling. It did seem such a pity that it all had to be make-believe, and that the age of wars between civilized nations had come to an end forever. If it had only been 100 years earlier what splendid times we should have had! Fancy being nineteen in 1793 with more than twenty years of war against Napoleon in front of one! However, all that was finished. The

British Army had never fired on white troops since the Crimea, and now the world was growing so sensible and pacific—and so democratic too—the great days were over.

Winston admired his father and identified with him in his career. He recalled that as a child he would see passers-by take off their hats in the streets and workmen grin when they saw his father's big moustache. It impressed him that everything his father said was reported in all the newspapers. For years Winston read every word his father publicly spoke and everything the newspapers said about him.

Shortly after Winston completed his course at Sandhurst, at age twenty, his father died. "All my dreams of comradeship with him, of entering Parliament at his side and in his support, were ended. There remained for me only to pursue his aims and vindicate his memory." Winston joined the Fourth Hussars Regiment.

This was the closing decade of the Victorian era, a time when the British Empire had enjoyed a long spell of almost unbroken peace. The opportunities to earn medals were becoming scarce. War service was held in high esteem and ardently sought by officers of every rank (Churchill 1930):

> . . . How we young officers envied the senior Major for his adventures. . . . How we admired the Colonel with his long row of decorations! We listened with almost insatiable interest to the accounts which they were good enough to give us on more than one occasion of stirring deeds and episodes already melting into the mist of time. How we longed to have a similar store of memories to unpack and display. . . . How we wondered whether our chance would ever come—whether we too in our turn would have battles to fight over again and again in the agreeable atmosphere of the after-dinner mess table? . . .
>
> This complaint was destined to be cured, and all our requirements were to be met to the fullest extent. The danger . . . which in those days seemed so real of Liberal and democratic governments making war impossible was soon to be proved illusory. . . . The little tidbits of fighting which the Indian frontier and the Sudan were soon to offer . . . were fiercely scrambled for throughout the British Army. But the South African War was to

attain dimensions which fully satisfied the needs of our small Army. And after that the deluge was still to come!

Winston Churchill wrote these last few paragraphs in 1930, as a fifty-six-year old man, looking back over his earlier life. The major portion of his career might have been behind him. The deluge to which he referred was World War I. The impending deluge of World War II was still a "gathering storm."

CASE 4: ADOLF

Adolf's father, the son of a poor cottager, "made something of himself " as a civil service worker. When he retired at age fifty-six, he bought a farm, which he worked himself. Adolf recalled:

It was at that time that the first ideals took shape in my breast . . . and though at that time I scarcely had any serious ideas as to the profession I should one day pursue, my sympathies were in any case not in the direction of my father's career.

Adolf found some books of a military nature in his father's library, including a popular edition concerning the Franco-German war (Hitler 1925):

It was not long before the great heroic struggle had become my greatest inner experience. From then on I became more and more enthusiastic about everything that was in any way connected with war or, for that matter, with soldiering.

His father decided that Adolf should become a civil servant. It was inconceivable to his father that Adolf might reject this. Thus, at age eleven, Adolf felt that he was forced into "opposition" for the first time in his life. The conflict with his father became even more difficult when, at age twelve, Adolf developed a plan of his own in opposition to his father's plan. He decided to become an artist. The consequences of this power struggle were "none too pleasant." Adolf's father has been described as a "veritable tyrant in his home" who would beat the children unmercifully and on one occasion beat Adolf so severely that he left the boy for dead (Langer 1972).

Adolf later considered that two outstanding facts were particularly significant as resulting from this period of conflict with his father:

First: *I became a nationalist.*
Second: *I learned to understand and grasp the meaning of history.*

Adolf remembered his adolescence as having been "an especially painful process." He felt that the question of his profession was decided more quickly than he had expected. When Adolf was thirteen, his father died. A few years later the death of his mother "put a sudden end to all my highflown plans."

Adolf was now "faced with the problem of somehow making my own living":

In my hand a suitcase full of clothes and underwear; in my heart an indomitable will, I journeyed to Vienna. I, too, hoped to wrest from Fate what my father had accomplished fifty years before; I, too, wanted to become "something"—but on no account a civil servant.

This was a difficult period for him. He believed that at this time his "eyes were opened" to the two "menaces" of Marxism and Jewry. Vienna represented "the living memory of the saddest period of my life." The world picture and philosophy which took shape within him then became "the granite foundation for all my acts."

Adolf recalled his reactions to the international climate of the time (Hitler 1925):

As a young scamp in my wild years, nothing had so grieved me as having been born at a time which obviously erected its Halls of Fame only to shopkeepers and government officials. The waves of historic events seemed to have grown so smooth that the future really seemed to belong only to the "peaceful contest of nations." . . . Why couldn't I have been born a hundred years earlier? Say at the time of the Wars of Liberation . . . I . . . regarded the period "of law and order" ahead of me as a mean and undeserved trick of Fate. . . .

The Boer War was like summer lightning to me. Every day I

waited impatiently for the newspapers and devoured dispatches and news reports, happy at the privilege of witnessing this heroic struggle even at a distance. The Russo-Japanese War found me considerably more mature, but also more attentive. . . . Since then many years have passed, and what as a boy had seemed to me a lingering disease, I now felt to be the quiet before the storm. . . . And then the first mighty lightning flash struck the earth; the storm was unleashed and with the thunder of Heaven there mingled the roar of the World War batteries. . . . To me those hours seemed like a release from the painful feelings of my youth.

Adolf quickly enlisted in a Bavarian regiment.

Adolf Hitler wrote the above paragraphs in 1924 at age thirty-five. The translator notes that even in this work Hitler was "fighting his persecutors, magnifying his person, creating a dream-world in which he can be an important figure." He was not yet The Leader.

Academia and Pseudo-Community

Dr. S. is a psychoanalyst whose recollections of the creation of a private society during his adolescence are quoted by Wolf et al. (1972) as an illustration of what they have termed an academia. They suggest that the creative formation of this special type of peer group can be involved with the reorganization of psychic structures which occurs during adolescence. The academia is viewed as a vehicle for those transformations of the self which lead to the internalization of a new stable ego ideal.

Gedo and Wolf (1973) focus on the role of idealization in the reorganization of the self which occurs in the adolescent process. They believe that Sigmund Freud entered adolescence still searching for idealized parental imagoes and that he found what he needed in the writing of Cervantes. Freud identified with Cervantes in his use of humor and wisdom concerning both the unworkable idealizations of his characters and his own grandiosity. Gedo and Wolf point to Cervantes's solution in *Don Quixote*. Freud perceived Part 1 as a comedy at the expense of childish reactions to the actualities of life. In Part 2, the hero ultimately learns to tolerate actuality and becomes "victorious over himself, which is the highest kind of victory." Victory over one's self does not mean the abandonment of ambitions or the surrender of high ideals but the capacity to see one's own ideals through a screen of wisdom and humor. Cervantes's road to victory over one's self involves the choice of an activity suited to one's talents and endowed with the perfection formerly reserved for the self.

In my initial study (Rothstein 1964), I coined the term "presidential assassination syndrome" to describe a constellation of factors which constituted a reasonably coherent syndrome, with those who threatened the president falling toward the less severe end of a continuum and the actual assassin falling at the more severe end. It was possible to formulate a "typical case" as an idealized composite picture. A basic element in such a prototype was confusion of identity. Typically, the subject would attempt to resolve his identity problems by military service. However, this attempt would prove unsuccessful. There would also be a frequent interest in other countries and other political ideologies such as Russia, communism, socialism, Marxism, Nazism, and so on. However, the subject clearly would have little real understanding of the position advocated and probably would have been disowned by the group. The subject would seem to feel that his act would be approved by some specific segment of society, making him a hero to that group. He would really be isolated and only wish to be a part of a group and would fantasize doing something spectacular to force recognition by the group. In reality, he would not be accepted by the group but only identify with it in his fantasy life. His expectations of approval from the group as a result of the act would be sadly disappointed (Rothstein 1964, 1965b, 1966, 1973, 1975).

Weinstein and Lyerly (1969) pointed out that threats to kill the president could be regarded "as attempts to form an emotional relationship, establish identity, and symbolize personal problems." They pointed out that many patients had used the language of politics and other institutions to give them a sense of identity and relate themselves in what Cameron has called a pseudo-community. Cameron (1943a, 1943b, 1959a, 1959b, 1967) had introduced the concept of the pseudo-community for the delusional group of persecutors created by a paranoid individual as an attempt at interpretation, anticipation, and validation of social behavior, and as a restitutive phenomenon.

In a previous paper (Rothstein 1975) I pointed out similarities and differences between the pseudo-community as applied by Weinstein and Lyerly and by me to the presidential assassination syndrome subjects, on the one hand, and the academia as described by Wolf et al., on the other. It appears that the pseudo-community may merely be a more pathological example of the same phenomenon as the academia.

The distinction can be quite blurred. In the paper just mentioned (Rothstein 1975), I purposely identified case 1 by his boyhood name, Tommy. If one did not realize that this was Woodrow Wilson, one might wonder whether the events described in his adolescence, such as the creation of an imaginary navy, were more akin to a pseudo-community than to an academia. Like Wilson's imaginary navy, Winston Churchill's imaginary army of soldiers which he commanded had aspects of a pseudo-community (as well as aspects of play) which blended into the academia of the "den." He, like Wilson, was apparently able to utilize these phenomena to assist him in finding an activity suited to his talents with a reasonable degree of conformity between internal and external reality.[1] He seemed to have been able to accept the strong input from his father, which did seem to correspond to a large extent to his own interests.

The pseudo-community aspect for Adolf Hitler seems to be somewhat more pronounced. He describes how the conflict with his father over finding an activity suited to his talents resulted in his becoming a fanatical nationalist and in his learning to "understand and grasp the meaning of history." This understanding and the meaning which he grasped seemed to have a delusional quality. The sad period in his life after the death of his parents and his rejection as a potential artist by the academy in Vienna "opened his eyes" to the "menaces" of Marxism and Jewry. Marxists and Jews had become negative pseudo-communities for him, in Cameron's sense.

Almost like patient G, described in a previous paper (Rothstein 1975), or like Oswald, Hitler had wished to start his own political party. Instead, shortly after World War I, he joined a small, newly formed, obscure, and weak party called the German Workers' party. His description of the early days of this party also sounds somewhat like Oswald's experiences with the Fair Play for Cuba party in New Orleans or the experiences of some of my other subjects.

Much as Wilson was drawn to change the structure of the clubs which he joined in college (Link 1966), Hitler changed the German Workers' party to meet his specifications. Shortly after joining, Hitler assumed leadership of the party, expelled the founder, Anton Drexler, and changed the name to the National Socialist German Workers' party and eventually to the National Socialist party (Hitler 1925; Stevens 1982).

The Army and the Adolescent Process

That is the miracle of our times: that you found me—
among so many millions! And that I found you is Germany's fortune! [HITLER (in Binion 1976)]

Whatever the psychological factors which led Hitler to develop in the way he did, the matter of understanding his personal development pales in comparison to the question of why the German people followed him. Leaders do govern by the consent of the governed. Hitler said that "what is essential will always be the inner accord between leader and multitude" (Binion 1976).

The events in the recent Falkland Islands crisis have dispelled any last remnants of belief that wars are caused solely by leaders and foisted on reluctant innocent populations. The populations of both countries enthusiastically endorsed prospects for military action, and it appeared that the leaders of neither Argentina nor Britain would have been able to remain in power if they had opposed the popular will.

The concepts of the academia and the pseudo-community can help us to understand the resonances between the leaders and the populations. But to these we must add another phenomenon—the army. I will use the term "army" to refer generically to all military organizations. The ready-made institution of the army can perform intrapsychic functions for those who are not so creative as to have an academia or so disturbed as to have a pseudo-community. Moreover, the army serves as the real-life counterpart, the prototype on which the creative person's academia may be modeled. Freud's *Academia Castellana* was modeled after Cervantes's satirical treatment of the profusion of pretentious successors to Plato's Academy which proliferated during the Renaissance (Gedo and Wolf 1973). Doctor S. modeled his mid-adolescent academia after literary and philosophical societies and modeled his earlier academia after boys' adventure stories (Wolf et al. 1972). Wilson's academia was modeled after a military organization, the British navy. Churchill's academia of toy soldiers and the "den" were modeled after a military organization, the British army. As with Dr. S.'s detective game, Churchill's academia had strong elements of play and games. At the other end of the scale, his academia blended into the reality of his actual military career. Hitler's pseudo-communities of malignant Jews and Marxists and his political party were strongly influenced by his interest in the Franco-German War and his experience in the German army during World War I. For Ron Kovic, the military provided a real model for childhood and adolescent games which blended into a sort of academia. But for him, as with a large portion of the population, the army served as a ready-made institution to "plug oneself into," without much modification of the institution into an individualized, unique phenomenon.

Wolf et al. (1972) suggest that the essence of adolescence, as they use the term, is the emergence of an inner necessity for new ideals, accompanied by opportunities encountered for such a transformation of the self. They believe this process is not universal but is fostered by cultures where changing conditions reinforce the desirability of wide departures from parental ideals or where change itself has been idealized. They see the academia as a means to maintain narcissistic balance while accomplishing the process of adolescence, a means utilized by the gifted individual whose change must be great.

"But what of more ordinary men? . . . The essential difference between ordinary and creative people is the distance between original ideals and the newly internalized ideals." They note that, for the majority of adolescents, heroes of sport or screen and occasionally historical figures usually provide models for the new idealizations. These authors felt that examination of ready-made adolescent groups was unrevealing because "Joining an already organized group is a public act; its private meaning is not discernible to observers and may, in fact, remain largely unconscious . . . the group hides the unconscious intentions of its members" (Wolf et al. 1972).

Utilizing the insights gained by these authors, however, one may view such a ready-made organization as the army and see that it performs a similiar function for the ordinary man. Ron Kovic's accounts clearly illustrate how playing soldier and planning on entering the marines influenced his ego ideal formation and his choice of an activity that he felt would be suited to his talents.

Wolf et al. (1972) describe how, with the aid of the academia, through his identification with the ideals of Cervantes, Freud set himself on the road to self-discovery, and how, in his idealization of Freud after his parents disappointed him, Dr. S. crystallized his future as a psychoanalyst. So, too, did Churchill's academia influence his future career, as did Hitler's pseudo-community academia. In a similar way, the army influenced Ron Kovic's choice of a career. On the other hand, the presidential assassination subjects tried but were not able to successfully utilize the army for their adolescent process. Even so, the army did have an influence on their psychological development and choice of symptoms.

It is notable to what extent recruiting material for the military services focuses on such matters as finding an activity suited to one's talents. An army ROTC booklet is entitled "Army ROTC: Be All You Can Be" (U.S. Army ROTC 1982). The U.S. Army Recruiting Command sends letters to high school seniors which advise, ". . . Whatever your abilities or interests—you'll find a skill to match; a skill that will give you an important job to do in the Army and in civilian life. . . . *The Army can help you meet your personal goals* . . . you'll have time to get to know the most important person in your future—you!" If the recipient requests further information, the army responds, "By sending for information, you've taken the first step toward making the most of your life . . . finding your special talents and skills."[2]

There is also a focus on ideals. A U.S. Marine Corps recruit training booklet (MC CLMPB 11051, undated) stresses the pride which the recruit will have in becoming a marine.

A U.S. Air Force (1979) applicant handout for officer training school (OTS) states that, for those who succeed in becoming officers, there is a great deal of pride, experience, and self-confidence, ". . . attributes that will enhance your opportunity to fulfill your goals and expectations. . . . Completing OTS and accepting a commission as an Air Force officer will mark a turning point in your life that will have few comparisons. . . . You will become a member of an elite group, charged with the awesome task of operating and managing the greatest assemblage of military power known to history. The task calls for dedication to an ideal and a sense of integrity that can accept no compromise."

A segment of the CBS television series "The Defense of the United States" (CBS News 1981) was quite relevant in this respect. Visiting an ICBM missile silo in North Dakota, the newsman, Bob Schieffer, asks the crewmen, "It must be an enormous responsibility . . . to be in charge, as you two gentlemen are, of the most powerful weapon . . . man has ever devised?" One of the crewmen answers: "Yes, sir, it is a definite challenge. It's more responsibility than I could obtain in a civilian world. And to me that is job satisfaction."

Internalization of Military Ideals

One is reminded that the job of the military is war and that war is violent. Today very few will speak for war, and even the military will claim that the job of the military is to keep the peace, albeit by preparing for war. Hitler was not bashful about his enthusiasm for war—not only during adolescence but also later. Churchill revealed his adolescent fascination with war and desire for combat but seems to indicate that he became wiser. Yet, even in his memoirs concerning World War II, he gives evidence of being exhilarated by war. Churchill writes of his August 1941 trip to North America: "On Sunday morning . . . Mr. Roosevelt came aboard H.M.S. *Prince of Wales* and . . . attended Divine Service on the quarterdeck . . . none who took part in it will forget the spectacle presented that sunlit morning on the crowded quarterdeck—I chose the hymns myself—'For Those in Peril on the Sea' and 'Onward Christian Soldiers.' We ended with 'O God, Our Help in Ages Past,' which Macauley reminds us the Ironsides had chanted. . . . Every word seemed to stir the heart. It was a great hour to live. Nearly half those who sang were soon to die" (Churchill 1950).

The ideals provided by the army are intimately related to war and violence. The 1895 Memorial Day speech entitled "The Soldier's Faith" given by Oliver Wendell Holmes clarifies this, as well as illustrating how the army, unlike the academia, serves to transmit ideals unchanged:

> . . . Now, at least, and perhaps as long as man dwells upon the globe, his destiny is battle, and he has to take the chances of war. . . . The ideals of the past for men have been drawn from war, as those for women have been drawn from motherhood. For all our prophecies, I doubt if we are ready to give up our inheritance. . . . To be a soldier or descended from soldiers, in time of peace to be ready to give one's life rather than to suffer disgrace, that is what the world has meant. . . .
>
> We do not save our traditions, in this country . . . It is the more necessary to learn the lesson afresh from perils newly sought, and perhaps it is not vain for us to tell the new generation what we learned in our day, and what we still believe. That the joy of life is living, is to put out all one's powers as far as they will go; that the measure of power is obstacles overcome; to ride boldly at what is in front of you, be it fence or enemy; to pray, not for comfort, but

for combat; to keep the soldier's faith against the doubts of civil life . . . to love glory more than the temptations of wallowing ease, but to know that one's final judge and only rival is oneself. . . . [Karsten 1980]

Wolf et al. (1972) and Gedo and Wolf (1973) describe how they believe that the period of adolescent change is a narcissistic peril in development and how the academia helps to maintain balance. They believe that the academia affords protection. It provides opportunity for the expression of regressively reactivated grandiosity which might be intolerably shameful if it were otherwise exposed. The dramatization involved may serve to discharge exhibitionistic pressure and appears to be helpful in the process of internalization of new structure. Other members of the group may help by serving such functions as mirrors, alter egos, and so on. The academia also assists in the de-idealization of the archaic imagoes, often by making the old imagoes seem ridiculous and also by explicitly espousing new values. The academia substitutes for the missing piece of internal structure which has been destroyed by the deidealization of the previously internalized parental imagoes. It lends cohesion to the self during the hiatus in self-guidance which exists until more workable guiding ideals have been set up.

The army and its activity, war, perform a similar function. Much as Ron Kovic admired the marines, he was surprised to find himself subjected to depreciation when he entered boot camp. The procedures at the New Cadet Barracks or "Beast Barracks" at West Point can be an ordeal for cadets which is one of the most traumatic experiences of their lives (Ellis and Moore 1974). Beast Barracks serves as an "intensive military indoctrination process." "The first week they rip you apart physically and then after that they start building you up again physically, but they are always tearing you down mentally." The reception and processing of new cadets on the traumatic first day, the tightly controlled schedule, and the rigorous and regimented training the cadets undergo during the first two months constitute ". . . a remarkably intensive and successful form of professional socialization . . . 'by which members of a profession learn the values, attitudes and behavior appropriate to their roles within the profession.' "

At the end of the process they are likely to agree with this cadet: "I have only been here two months. I am not yet a member of the Corps, but the feeling of Duty, Honor, and Country has already begun to build in me. I know now why Patton, MacArthur, and other men like them have given so much to their country. It is because West Point has instilled in them a faith in God and in our country that overrules all other feelings. . ." (Ellis and Moore 1974).

The process of removing the old ideals and replacing them with new ones is apparently intentionally fostered by the army, sometimes approaching the concept of brainwashing. The following description of officer training also clarifies the purpose of boot camp for enlisted men:

> Officer candidates are subjected to intensive training, a great part of which is directed toward molding a man's social attitudes to conform to the traditional stereotypes of the officer. . . . The hopeful candidate is now subjected to a nearly catastrophic experience which breaks down to a large extent his previous personality organization. His previous valuations fail him and in order to find a basis for self-respect, he must adopt new standards or escape from the field. At the same time new, appropriate attitudes are built up and established. The catastrophic experience provides a kind of purgatory, a definite demarcation from the candidate's enlisted incarnation that puts a barrier between the new officer and his enlisted memories. It has some of the characteristics of a conversion experience, or the ordeal of the medieval knight. . . . Aside from constituting a frontal attack on any civilian residue in the candidate's personality, these practices also involve the learning of new habits and values. [Stouffer et al. 1949]

Violence is intimately involved with these new habits and values, even though often superficially screened. Janowitz (1960) described the role of "honor" as the basis of the belief system of the military establishment: "When military honor is effective, its coercive power is considerable, since it persistently points to a single overriding directive: The professional soldier always fights." He notes that military honor has been redefined away from aristocratic forms venerating the martial spirit to the practical justification of military ideals and quotes S. L. A. Marshall: "Military ideals are not different than the ideals which make any man sound in himself and in his relation to others. . . . Every normal man needs to have some sense of a contest, some feeling of a resistance to overcome before he can make the best use of his faculties."

Instead of glorifying war, as do the speeches of Oliver Wendell

Holmes, the writings of Adolf Hitler, and even the memoirs of Winston Churchill to some extent, the military has developed a sense of honor "rooted in the practical contributions of the profession rather than in the survival of feudal notions of military glory" (Janowitz 1960). However, the sober-minded approach represented above and in current recruiting literature may mask the underlying grandiosity that can still be an important motivating factor.

War and the Self

War is the perfect stage on which to act out archaic grandiosity—a domain in which it can in fact be lived out. The academia may provide secrecy or privacy which permits a safe degree of exposure for grandiosity. The army provides a social structure which validates grandiosity, and war provides a habitat in which one can live out the grandiosity. As Oliver Wendell Holmes recalled in another speech, "There is . . . a something more exalting, more ethereal, more word escaping than even our memories—a something . . . in which I would sum up what the war did for our souls. It is the romantic spirit. It is the fire of life. Those who have not known what it is to march straight to where you see the bullets striking may talk . . . about the trials of civil life. . . . But the men who have been soaked in a sea of death and who somehow have survived, have got something from it which has transfigured their world. . . . They know the passion of life and the irony of fate" (Karsten 1980).

It is probably the fact that violence in war so effectively permits and fosters this grandiosity that gives it such an appeal in identity formation.

Gray (1970) writes of the "quality of excitement scarcely experienced before or since" resulting from battle experiences such as the landing on D-Day, living through an air raid, and so on. "In such an emotional situation there is often a surge of vitality and a glimpse of potentialities of what we really are or have been or might become, as fleeting as it is genuine." He notes that the experience of communal effort in battle has been for many veterans a high point in their lives, "the one great lyric passage in their lives." He describes a feeling of power and liberation. "We feel earnest and gay at such moments because we are liberated from our individual impotence and are drunk with the power that union with our fellows brings. . . . There is something more and equally important. The sense of power and liberation that comes over men at such moments stems from a source beyond the union of men. I believe it is nothing less than the assurance of immortality that makes self-sacrifice at these moments so relatively easy.''

A British veteran of war in Burma and the Crimea later wrote, ''That 'war is a horrible thing,' is a very nice heading for the page of a schoolgirl's copybook, but I confess that in my heart I always thoroughly enjoyed it. . . . It is only through experience of the sensation that we learn how intense, even in anticipation, is the rapture-giving delight which the attack upon an enemy affords. I cannot analyze nor weigh, nor can I justify the feeling. But once experienced, all other subsequent sensations are but as a tinkling of a doorbell in comparison with the throbbing of Big Ben'' (Farwell 1981).

It might be argued that views such as these are either remnants of a bygone era or the productions of aberrant individuals. Hitler may have been an aberrant individual, but a whole nation followed him. Churchill was hardly an aberrant individual. His youth may have been in a bygone era, but similar feelings show up in his memoirs of World War II, and his role in the perfection of terror bombing in that war has provided us with the most likely scenario for World War III. It seems to me that our current fashion to deplore war has led us to disavow, deny, and even repress awareness of feelings such as those referred to above, much as the Victorians dealt with sexuality. We need to recognize and face these feelings and attitudes in order to penetrate the screen of rationalizations which currently perpetuate militarism.

Archaic grandiosity is, of course, unrealistic. Many soldiers are killed. Many others, like Ron Kovic, are seriously wounded physically, which puts an end to the grandiosity as well as to the realistic development of much of their potential. Others are overwhelmed psychologically. Erikson (1968) speaks of men whose ego identity throve in military service but sometimes broke down after discharge because ''the war had provoked them into more ambitious self-images than their more restricted peacetime identities could afford to sustain.''

At the same time that war can destroy identity and the self, it can force a different organization of identity and of the self. Gray (1970) tells of reading in a German newspaper, taken from a prisoner, a letter from a soldier who had been on the Russian front for long years, who lamented that the war had robbed him of any sense of self-identity and that he no longer possessed an ego and a personal fate. But Gray describes a corresponding expansion of the self: ''We are able to disregard personal danger at such moments by transcending the self, by forgetting our separateness . . . the self is no longer important to the observer; it is absorbed into the objects with which it is concerned." The ecstatic experience is "a state of being outside the self . . . breaking down of the barriers of the self."

Many will not be able to tolerate these extremes, but the experiences have an effect on those who survive them, on others whom the survivors influence, and in the institutions such as the army designed to perpetuate these traditions. Erikson (1968) notes, "As a historical focus of many part-identifications the military identity thus continues to be dominant unconsciously even in those who are excluded from its consummation by political developments."

Like the academia, the army and war can substitute for or cover a gap in the internal psychic structure. Gray (1970) states that in war "we feel rescued from the emptiness with us. For losing ourselves we gain a relationship to something greater than the self. . . ." He describes a conversation with a Frenchwoman who had suffered during the war but was now living comfortably. She confessed with great earnestness that, despite everything, those earlier times had been more satisfying than the present. "My life is so unutterably boring nowadays. . . . I do not love war or want to return. But at least it made me feel alive, as I have not felt alive before or since." He was also told something similar by a German friend. He concluded, "Peace exposed a void in them that war's excitement had enabled them to keep covered up. . . . Violence has been, I think, a perennial refuge from this painful malady."

Individual Identity and the Nation

Erikson (1950) proposes that national unity can become "a matter of the preservation of identity, and thus a matter of (human) life and death, far surpassing the question of political systems." He writes that "men . . . need to feel that they are of some special kind (tribe or nation, class or caste, family, occupation, or type) whose insignia they will wear with vanity and conviction, and defend . . . against the foreign, the inimical, the not-so-humankinds" (Erikson 1968).

Frantz Fanon (1963) spoke of violence of "national liberation." He said that for colonized people the violence of decolonization invests their characters with positive and creative qualities. "The practice of violence binds them together as a whole. . . . In the same way . . . the

55

building-up of the nation, is helped on by the existence of this cement which has been mixed with blood and anger." In his introduction to Fanon's book, Jean-Paul Sartre goes even further: "Make no mistake about it; by this mad fury . . . by their ever-present desire to kill us . . . they have become men . . . this irrepressible violence . . . is man recreating himself . . . the native cures himself of colonial neurosis by thrusting out the settler through force of arms. When his rage boils over, he rediscovers his lost innocence and he comes to know himself in that he himself creates his self."

Grinker[3] has illustrated the concept of identity by recalling an experience when he was in the army during World War II. On an occasion when the troops were gathered together for some purpose such as seeing a visiting entertainer, he, looking over this large massive gathering, suddenly had a vivid perception which highlighted a simultaneous awareness of his own unique individuality and his being part of a larger group endeavor. He described this as the most distinct and powerful experience of his own identity that he could recall. He noted how it illustrated the two complementary aspects of identity, the uniqueness of the individual and the continuity with the larger group.

Grinker and Spiegel (1963) wondered about the motivation for combat: "What is the force that compels a man to risk his life day after day, to endure the constant tension, the fear of death . . . the sight of the injured, the bleeding, the dying. . . . What drives him to dump four thousand pounds of death on the little people in the factories miles below him? What can possess a rational man to make him act so irrationally?" They note that the men did not have a clear comprehension of the political reasons for the war. Instead, feelings of identification with the group, largely unconscious, were more important motivating factors.

Erikson (1968) has postulated crises of development at various points of the life cycle, with the crisis of identity formation being the essence of the adolescent phase of the life cycle. He notes that creative individuals may resolve such crises by offering to their contemporaries a new model of resolution, expressed in works of art or in original deeds. In general, for most, "the social institution which is the guardian of identity is what we have called *ideology*. . . . For it is through their ideology that social systems enter into the fiber of the next generation and attempt to absorb into their lifeblood the rejuvenated power of youth." A failure of this process leads to *"identity confusion."* He discusses how various *"part symptoms"* of such confusion may relate to antecedents in childhood. He also suggests ways in which the social process attempts to deal with such *part symptoms*. The army appears repeatedly in these solutions.

A regression to the early stage of infancy can lead to "time confusion." The adolescent may not trust time. Every delay may appear to be a deceit, every wait an experience of impotence, every hope a danger, every plan a catastrophe, and every possible provider a potential traitor. One solution may be "goose stepping to blaring trumpets in preparation for the Thousand Year Reich."

There may be "self-consciousness" dating back to the original doubt which concerned the trustworthiness of the parents in early childhood. A societal phenomenon corresponding to this second conflict is a "universal trend toward some form of uniformity either in special uniforms or in distinctive clothing through which incomplete self certainty, for a time, can hide in group certainty." The army can provide this.

There may be a *"role fixation"* in connection with earlier conflicts between free initiative and oedipal guilt. Social institutions may attempt to deal with this by combining "some badge or sacrifice or submission with an energetic push toward sanctioned ways of action. . . . This special proclivity—namely, the achievement of a sense of free choice as the very result of ritual regimentation—is, of course, universally utilized in Army life."

There may be *"work paralysis"* as a logical sequence of a sense of inadequacy of one's general equipment dating back to school age. It may not reflect a lack of potential as much as unrealistic demands "made by an ego ideal willing to settle only for omnipotence or omniscience . . . young people must have learned to enjoy a sense of *apprenticeship* . . . in order not to need the thrill of destruction."

"Social institutions support the strength and distinctiveness of the budding work identity by offering those who are still learning and experimenting a certain status of *apprenticeship,* a moratorium characterized by defined duties and sanctioned competitions as well as by special license." The army can provide both the apprenticeship and the thrill of destruction.

There are also aspects of identity formation which anticipate future development. Although Erikson does not cite it as explicitly, the army seems to represent one of society's ways of shaping these developments.

There is a need to form a *"polarization of sexual differences"* rather than *"bisexual confusion."* The army has in the past traditionally been a male organization, fostering its concept of "masculinity." There may develop changes in this function since women are now admitted into the army. However, the United States does not yet seem ready to accept women as subjects for military draft and certainly not as combatants.

There is a need to learn to take "leadership" as well as to assume *followership* and avoid "authority confusion." A "common 'cause' permits others to follow and to obey (and the leader himself to obey higher leaders) and thus to replace the parent images set up in the infantile superego with the hierarchy of leader-images inhabiting the available gallery of ideals. . . ." Leadership and followership are essential aspects of the army.

The final need is to develop an ideological commitment rather than a confusion of values. The army plays a role in that area also.

Conclusions

To answer the questions posed at the beginning of the chapter: Yes, it is true that people can and do use violence to solve their identity crises. Violence, as discussed here, contributes by its pervasive influence in the institution of the army. The army serves for many "ordinary men" a function similar to that described by Wolf et al. (1973) for the academia. That is, it assists in maintaining narcissistic balance and facilitates the transformation of the self characteristic of adolescence. Unlike the academia, however, the army tends to transmit social values unchanged. In addition, the army influences the form of the academia for many creative individuals destined to become leaders. As a result, there is a natural resonance between the leaders and the population at large. Erikson (1963) notes that "in Germany, then, we saw a highly organized and highly educated nation surrender to the imagery of ideological adolescence."

Since the job of the army is war, the values and ideals which it transmits for society from one generation to another are strongly influenced by war and thus act to perpetuate this social institution. Even in democratic societies which desire peace, it has not been possible to totally avoid this resonance between leader and population that has a warlike quality. Erikson (1968) remarks on how the "world struggle . . . makes a military identity a part of young adulthood in peacetime."

How does violence contribute to identity formation? The release of archaic grandiosity in battle and the comradeship and bonding seem to have a powerful influence. The perception that the self has been expanded, whether illusory or realistic, is seductive and long remembered in a positive light. This has an effect not only on those who experience it but also on those who hear of their exploits and shape their ambitions and ideals after the same models.

War performs a function for society indirectly through the effect of the army and more directly by providing a structure which fills an intrapsychic void for many. Much as we deplore the deleterious effect of the present Cold War with its arms race and its threat of nuclear annihilation, we should not overlook the likelihood that for many (both hawks and doves) it is probably a major point of orientation in their lives. Much of the opposition to rational efforts toward arms control (let alone disarmament) represents an effort to cling to the structure provided by the Cold War because of an emptiness within.

We may end on a more encouraging note. There are also strong psychological forces operating against violence and killing. Social effort seems to be required to overcome this individual inhibition. S. L. A. Marshall (in Karsten 1980) was distressed to find how few soldiers in combat actually fired their weapons. In various situations only fifteen to twenty-five men out of a hundred would take any part with their weapons, even in the face of great danger.

Karsten (1968) describes that

. . . social scientists accompanying numerous American combat units in both theaters of World War II found that only about one in every five soldiers with individually operated weapons actually fired his weapon, and that this was so even during intense fire fights or when they were confronted with visible targets. Men who had to join together with others to fire weapons (machine gunners, artillery men), displayed no such reluctance to fire, in part because they were drawn into the act by primary-group pressures. In like fashion, at Gettysburg over 18,000 muskets were found on the battlefield with unmistakable evidence that their owners had not fired them at anyone that day; 12,000 of them had two charges, neither of which had been discharged, rammed down the barrel; 6,000 more had from three to ten such charges, and another had no fewer than 23 charges! Some men had probably simply panicked and were loading their weapons purposelessly. But others were probably loading quite deliberately, in order to give the *appearance* that they were firing.

Marshall is interested in rewarding those who do fire and in overcoming the resistance in the others to the extent possible, including encouraging a habit of free firing in combat. Perhaps this approach contributed to the character of the Vietnam War with its "free fire zones." I recall seeing news clips early in the Vietnam War, showing how we Americans were trying to teach reluctant Vietnamese soldiers to fight—and most of all to persuade them to want to fight. I recall thinking that perhaps they should be giving us the lessons.

Perhaps we do not have to counteract a supposedly warlike "human nature" in order to counteract war. Perhaps what we need to do is to diminish those social influences which act against the individual inhibition and reluctance to kill. It may be hoped that, if there is such resistance to using weapons to kill, maybe humankind will yet refrain from using our nuclear arsenal.

NOTES

1. Also see Kohut 1966.
2. William S. Graf, undated form letter; Graf, personal letter, February 14, 1982.
3. Roy R. Grinker, personal communication, 1961.

REFERENCES

Binion, R. 1976. *Hitler among the Germans*. New York: Elsevier.

Cameron, N. 1943a. The paranoid pseudo-community. *American Journal of Sociology* 49:32–38.

Cameron, N. 1943b. The development of paranoid thinking. *Psychological Review* 50:219–233.

Cameron, N. 1959a. The paranoid pseudo-community revisited. *American Journal of Sociology* 65:52–58.

Cameron, N. 1959b. Paranoid conditions and paranoia. In S. Arieti, ed. *American Handbook of Psychiatry*. Vol. 1. New York: Basic.

Cameron, N. 1967. Psychotic disorders. II: Paranoid reactions. In

A. M. Freedman and H. I. Kaplan, eds. *Comprehensive Textbook of Psychiatry*. Baltimore: Williams & Wilkins.

CBS News. 1981. "CBS Reports: The Defense of the United States." Broadcast June 14, 15, 16, 17, 18.

Churchill, R. S. 1966. *Winston S. Churchill*. Vol. 1, *Youth: 1874–1900*. Cambridge: Riverside; Boston: Houghton Mifflin.

Churchill, W. S. 1930. *My Early Life: A Roving Commission*. New York: Scribner's, 1958.

Churchill, W. S. 1950. *The Second World War: The Grand Alliance*. New York: Bantam, 1962.

Donovan, R. J. 1964. *The Assassins*. New York: Popular.

Ellis, J., and Moore, R. 1974. *School for Soldiers: West Point and the Profession of Arms*. New York: Oxford University Press.

Erikson, E. H. 1950. *Childhood and Society*. 2d ed. New York: Norton, 1963.

Erikson, E. H. 1968. *Identity, Youth and Crisis*. New York: Norton.

Fanon, F. 1963. *The Wretched of the Earth*. New York: Grove.

Farwell, B. 1981. *Mr. Kipling's Army: All the Queen's Men*. New York: Norton.

Gedo, J. E., and Wolf, E. S. 1973. Freud's *Novelas Ejemplares*. *Annual of Psychoanalysis* 1:299–317.

Givens, R., and Nettleship, A., eds. 1976. Discussions on war and human aggression. In S. Tax, ed. *World Anthropology*. The Hague: Mouton.

Gray, J. 1970. *The Warriors: Reflections on Men in Battle*. New York: Harper Colophon.

Grinker, R. R., and Spiegel, J. P. 1963. *Men under Stress*. New York: McGraw-Hill.

Hitler, A. 1925. *Mein Kampf*. Translated by R. Manheim. Boston: Houghton Mifflin, 1971.

Janowitz, M. 1960. *The Professional Soldier: A Social and Political Portrait*. Glencoe, Ill.: Free Press.

Karsten, P. 1978. *Soldiers and Society: The Effects of Military Service and War on American Life*. Westport, Conn.: Greenwood.

Karsten, P., ed. 1980. *The Military in America: From the Colonial Era to the Present*. New York: Free Press.

Kohut, H. 1966. Forms and transformations of narcissism. *Journal of the American Psychoanalytic Association* 14:243–272.

Kovic, R. 1976. *Born on the Fourth of July*. New York: Pocket Books.

Langer, W. C. 1972. *The Mind of Adolf Hitler: The Secret Wartime Report.* New York: Basic.

Link, A. S. 1966. *The Papers of Woodrow Wilson.* Vol. 1, *1856–1880.* Princeton, N.J.: Princeton University Press.

President's Commission on the Assassination of President Kennedy. 1964. *Report.* Washington, D.C.: Government Printing Office.

Rothstein, D. A. 1964. Presidential assassination syndrome. *Archives of General Psychiatry* 11:245–254.

Rothstein, D. A. 1965a. Presidential assassination syndrome: further studies. Paper read at the University of North Carolina, Chapel Hill, March 26.

Rothstein, D. A. 1965b. Presidential assassination syndrome. Paper read at 121st Annual Meeting of the American Psychiatric Association. New York, May 6.

Rothstein, D. A. 1966. Presidential assassination syndrome: II, application to Lee Harvey Oswald. *Archives of General Psychiatry* 15:260–266.

Rothstein, D. A. 1968a. Information and conclusions presented to the National Commission on the Causes and Prevention of Violence (Eisenhower Commission), Task Force on Political Assassination. Washington, D.C., October 3.

Rothstein, D. A. 1968b. The assassin and the assassinated—as non-patient subjects of psychiatric investigation. Preliminary version, read at Midwest Regional Meeting on Violence and Aggression of American Psychiatric Association and American Medical Association, Chicago, November 15.

Rothstein, D. A. 1971a. The president as person and public figure. Chairman's introductory remarks for special session at the 124th annual meeting of the American Psychiatric Association, Washington, D.C., May 4.

Rothstein, D. A. 1971b. The assassin and the assassinated—as non-patient subjects of psychiatric investigation. In J. Fawcett, ed. *Dynamics of Violence.* Chicago: American Medical Association.

Rothstein, D. A. 1971c. Presidential assassination syndrome: a psychiatric study of the threat, the deed, and the message. In W. J. Crotty, ed. *Assassinations and the Political Order.* New York: Harper & Row.

Rothstein, D. A. 1973. Reflections on a contagion of assassination. *Life-threatening Behavior* 3:105–130.

Rothstein, D. A. 1975. On presidential assassination: the academia and the pseudo-community. *Adolescent Psychiatry* 4:264–298.

Stevens, W. L. 1982. "On warfare." Tape recorded supplement to book. Chicago: City College of Chicago.

Stouffer, S. A.; Lumsdaine, A. A.; Lumsdaine, M. H.; Williams, R. M., Jr.; Smith, M. B.; Janis, I. L.; Star, S. A.; and Cottrell, L. S., Jr. 1949. *Studies in Social Psychology in World War II. The American Soldier.* Vol. 2, *Combat and Its Aftermath.* Princeton, N.J.: Princeton University Press.

Stouffer, S. A.; Suchman, E. A.; DeVinney, L. C.; Star, S. A.; and Williams, R. M., Jr. 1949. *Studies in Social Psychology in World War II. The American Soldier.* Vol. 1, *Adjustment during Army Life.* Princeton, N.J.: Princeton University Press.

U.S. Air Force. 1979. ATC FM 1305-HO. *Applicant Handout— Officer Training School (OTS), USAF.* Washington, D.C.: Government Printing Office.

U.S. Army ROTC. 1982. *Be All You Can Be: Four Year Scholarship Application Packet School Year 1982–83.*

U.S. Marine Corps. Undated. MC CLMPB 11051. *Marine Corps Recruit Training for Men.*

Weinstein, E. A., and Lyerly, O. G. 1969. Symbolic aspects of presidential assassination. *Psychiatry* 32:1–11.

Wolf, E. S.; Gedo, J. E.; and Terman, D. M. 1972. On the adolescent process as a transformation of the self. *Journal of Youth and Adolescence* 1:257–272.

6 COMPETENT ADOLESCENTS FROM DIFFERENT SOCIOECONOMIC AND ETHNIC CONTEXTS

JOHN G. LOONEY AND JERRY M. LEWIS

Introduction

The view that normal adolescent development is characterized by turmoil, disruption, and maladaptive behavior (Blos 1962; Erickson 1956; Freud 1958; Hall 1904; Josselyn 1954; Lindemann 1964; Spiegel 1961) has been challenged by studies of nonclinical samples (Douvan and Adelson 1966; Looney and Gunderson 1978; Masterson 1967; Mead 1928, 1930; Offer 1969; Oldham 1978; Weiner and Del Gaudio 1976). These more recent studies emphasized the dangers of extrapolating from clinical samples and suggest that, although situational anxiety and brief episodes of depressive affect may occur, serious symptomatic behavior in adolescents is not part of the modal developmental experience.

Blotcky and Looney (1980) have pointed out the need for empirical studies of nonclinical samples of adolescents from other than white, middle-class populations and have emphasized the need to assess the impact of family variables on adolescent development.

This is a preliminary report based on the unique opportunity to compare two groups of adolescents: those from white, middle-, and upper-middle-class families and those from black, working-class families. Its particular focus will be on adolescents judged to be functioning at good or superior levels of adjustment.

JOHN G. LOONEY AND JERRY M. LEWIS

Method

In the late 1960s Lewis, Beavers, Gossett, and Phillips (1976) studied well-functioning families and the individuals who constitute them. Forty-four intact, white, middle- and upper-middle-class families containing adolescents were studied. Although no individuals in the study had been in legal difficulty or psychiatric treatment during the two years preceding data collection, family competence[1] was found to vary across a broad range of functioning.

Twelve years later the study was replicated on a group of eighteen lower-income, working-class, intact black families containing adolescents. Both samples were studied with a variety of techniques, including family interviews, family interactional testing, home visits, individual exploratory interviews, and a large number of paper-and-pencil tests. Data from families and individuals were collected and evaluated independently in order to avoid contamination of ratings.

The particular focus of this study are those adolescents judged to be functioning at good or superior levels of psychological adjustment. The basic research question is—What are the similarities and differences in these two groups of adolescents who come from such very different socioeconomic and ethnic contexts?

The data to be reported in this paper are derived from the semi-structured, exploratory interviews of twenty-two adolescents accomplished by clinicians with broad clinical and research experience.[2]

The interviews were designed to explore the subject's capacity for work, play, and love. Work was evaluated by exploring the individual's involvement in school, extracurricular activities, outside employment, and tasks at home. Play was evaluated by exploring the subject's use of leisure time. Love was evaluated by probing the individual's relationships with friends, family members, and intimates. The interview transcripts were rated on a five-point Life Adaptation Scale based on the work, play, and love criteria. Satisfactory interrater reliabilities were obtained in both studies (Pearsonian $r = .48, P < .025$ in the initial study, and .49 to .64, $P < .01$ in the second study).[3]

In the initial study nineteen adolescents were interviewed, and eleven of those who received good or superior ratings are contrasted with the eleven of thirty-seven adolescents receiving comparable ratings in the second study (sixteen of the thirty-seven were rated as functioning at "average" levels of adaptation and ten at poor levels).

At the time of data collection, the adolescents from the initial sample had an average age of fifteen years. Those from the second sample had an average of 15.8 years.

Findings

The findings can be described from the perspective of eleven areas of functioning. These are:

1. Personal relationship skills as demonstrated toward the interviewer (warmth, openness).

2. Ability to describe one's self and to understand one's own complex needs and motivations.

3. Active/passive orientation.

4. Educational achievements and aspirations.

5. Extracurricular activities.

6. Work.

7. Future orientation.

8. General social relationships.

9. Heterosexual relationships.

10. Attitudes toward parents and family.

11. Problems with authority, legal problems, substance usage.

PERSONAL RELATIONSHIP SKILLS

Individuals in both groups of adolescents demonstrated warmth toward the interviewer and related to him with an openness and easy-going manner which clinicians do not observe often in patient populations. In both groups, the young people appeared to be secure in their sense of self. This self-security was particularly intriguing in the black adolescents because several in this group commented they had never had a comparable interview with a white adult.

ABILITY TO DESCRIBE SELF

Teenagers in both of these groups demonstrated some ability to describe themselves in terms of complex needs, drives, aspirations, and motivations. Again, this ability is in stark contrast to that which the clinician usually observes with patients. There was some difference, however, between the two groups. The black adolescents were less likely to describe themselves in terms as three-dimensional as were the white teenagers. In particular, the white teenagers seemed to be gaining mastery in understanding the difference between their own desires and societal and parental expectations. The black adolescents seemed to have greater difficulty in separating their desires from parental expectations.

ACTIVE/PASSIVE ORIENTATION

It was clear that individuals in both groups were active, assertive youngsters. They were doers. As will be noted, they were involved in a wide variety of activities.

EDUCATIONAL ACHIEVEMENTS AND ASPIRATIONS

Teenagers in both these groups were good students. Average grades were uncommon. Honor roll performance was common. There was, however, a subtle difference with regard to attitudes toward school. The black youngsters conceptualized education as the pathway out of lower-income status. These youngsters often utilized the most advanced programs the public school system offered. For example, a majority of them were either in honors programs or attending magnet schools (high schools with specialized curricula for various vocational directions). They were proud of their schools. One youngster said, about his almost all-black high school:

> It's a great school if you want to learn. . . . All of the other schools, they usually down on Carver High, but after they transfer and come over there, then they see how it really is. And most people . . . well, we had the Governor come over once and he couldn't believe it was Carver—you know, no people in the halls and no paper laying in the halls, no writing on the walls, around the school was clean and the wind didn't pick up and blow trash around. Other than that, they was shocked to know this was really Carver and we're striving to come from the bottom up.

Of his aspirations in life, one young black male said:

> Ten years? I will be . . . let's see . . . I plan to be living in Dallas. . . . I don't know if I will be married or not. I ain't thought about that. But, I don't know. . . . I plan to have a good job, you

know. So, I plan to be . . . I plan to be somebody. . . . I'm talking about somebody you know. Worth something . . . popular . . . that's what I want to be. Somebody.

The adolescent went on to relate his goals to the need to use the school
system to achieve them.

The white adolescents, while being good students, seemed to take
for granted that they were headed for college. Often they expressed
some degree of boredom about school or uncertainty that education
was necessarily the only pathway to their aspirations.

EXTRACURRICULAR ACTIVITIES

Adolescents in both of these groups were involved in a wide variety
of extracurricular activities. They served on student councils, as presi-
dents and members of clubs, in honor societies, and on athletic teams.
There was little difference between the level of extracurricular activities in both groups. One minor difference was that the black girls
participated more in athletic activities than did their white age-mates.

WORK

There was a marked difference in the amount of compensated work
done by youngsters in these two groups. The white adolescents tended
to think of work in terms of tasks around the house. The black adolescents performed fewer of these kinds of chores, but almost all of them
were involved in paid part-time jobs.

FUTURE ORIENTATION

Youngsters in both groups were oriented toward the future. When
asked what their lives would be like in five or ten years, they articulated responses which seemed reasonable in terms of their abilities and
ambitions. The white adolescents were more prone to assume that the
future would work out well because the past had. The black adolescents, on the other hand, did not assume that a successful future would
come as a matter of course. Rather consistently, they articulated a
combination of attributes that would lead to a successful future, and
these were: honesty, hard work, the ability to get along with people,
education, and achievement. Adolescents in both groups aspired to

join the ranks of people in respected job roles. Many of the white adolescents wanted to be doctors, lawyers, scientists, or entrepreneurs. Most of the youngsters in the black group, however, aspired to occupational niches that were clearly above those of their parents but not necessarily in the professional ranks.

GENERAL SOCIAL RELATIONSHIPS

Adolescents in both of these groups had wide circles of acquaintances. Apparently these teenagers were respected by, and popular with, their peers. In both groups, the importance of one or two close, same-sex friends was stated. One subtle difference was that the black adolescents made statements suggesting they were more particular in defining their close friends. This discriminating quality was in response to their views that the modal adolescent in their social and educational milieu was not headed for the same success to which they aspired.

HETEROSEXUAL RELATIONSHIPS

In the area of heterosexual relationships, there was a major difference. Youngsters in the white group tended to begin serious interest in the opposite sex at about the time car dating was possible (age sixteen). None of the black adolescents in this group had, or planned to have, an automobile. Their heterosexual interest began earlier, for both boys and girls. Almost half had had intercourse with several partners by the time of the interview. Those who had not, discussed intense peer pressure to experience it. Although most of the white adolescents had had "going steady" relationships, none had had intercourse.

ATTITUDE TOWARD PARENTS

Adolescents in both groups had positive feelings toward both parents. In both groups there was a slight inclination to view the mother as the parent to whom they were closer and with whom they could more easily discuss sensitive topics. In both groups the father was more likely to be seen as the disciplinarian.

One interesting similarity between youngsters in these two groups is that they commonly saw their parents as stricter than the parents of their peers. Although they complained occasionally about this strictness, they felt that rules and discipline were fair and that an authoritative assuredness on the part of their parents was a source of their own and their family's strength. One of the white youngsters stated:

> Well, and I'm kinda, I'm pretty glad that they are strict because people that, I mean like some of the people I know, they don't have strict parents, they're bad and things like that, and it doesn't affect them if they ground them and stuff like that.

PROBLEMS WITH AUTHORITY, LEGAL PROBLEMS, SUBSTANCE USAGE

None of the youngsters had any significant conflicts with authority. One or two in each group had been sent to the principal's office for minor transgressions in school but, on balance, they were well behaved. None had any legal difficulty. With regard to substance usage, approximately one-third of the white adolescents had drunk beer on several occasions. One of the black adolescents had tried marijuana once. Consistently, however, in both groups drug usage was seen as necessitating association with people they did not like or trust, unnecessary for fun, and potentially destructive to their future.

In review, teenagers from these two research groups separated in time by twelve years, many thousands of dollars of family income, neighborhood, and color of skin demonstrated some differences but were much more similar than they were different. Adolescents from both groups were outgoing, warm, and person oriented. They had high energy levels and manifested high levels of initiative. They seemed secure in their evolving sense of self, comfortable in their family relationships, and confident about the future. At a different level of observation, their psychological mechanisms were either mature or, at worst, neurotic; there was no evidence of immature or primitive defenses (Vaillant 1977). Symptoms of significant anxiety, depression, or behavior disorder were absent. As a group, the twenty-two youngsters appeared to be traversing adolescence with little turmoil.

Discussion

The data from the exploratory interviews of adolescents rated as functioning at above-average levels of adaptation document that the two groups are much more alike than different. This finding seems all the more striking in view of the pronounced socioeconomic differences between the two groups. The design of the study of working-class black families called for the inclusion of only intact families. The average total family income for the eighteen families was $11,080, with a range of $6,600–$15,000. This contrasts with a national average for all two-parent, black families in which both parents work of approximately $22,000 (*Dallas Morning News* 1981). Another way of locating this group of families within the range of socioeconomic factors is to note that, on the average, the families were only slightly more than $3,000 above the size-adjusted family poverty level.[4]

Another way of emphasizing the different socioeconomic contexts of these two groups of youngsters is the neighborhoods in which they live. The white adolescents lived in an affluent suburb with large brick homes, landscaped yards, and at least two cars in the garage. The black adolescents lived in an inner-city area of modest frame homes interspersed with shacks, many of the yards filled with junk, and, most often, one old car parked on the street.

Although we do not know all of the factors that account for the similar patterns of high levels of adaptation in these two groups, our data suggest one factor we wish to emphasize. The adolescents came from families that were much alike in terms of their organizational structure, methods of communicating, openness with affect, and problem-solving efficiency. Despite the clear socioeconomic and ethnic differences, the families of both groups of adolescents were the types of small social systems that encourage the development of autonomy and provide a strong sense of emotional support and human connectedness. One index of this finding is the global level of family competence as rated independently from family interactional testing. On a ten-point family competence scale (1, most competent; 10, severely dysfunctional), the families of the white adolescents had an average rating of 3.8, and the families of the black adolescents an average of 3.6.[5] Both groups of adolescents, therefore, had the good fortune to be members of families rated as very competent.

No systematic attempt was made in this study to elucidate significant differences between boys and girls in regard to such things as type of extracurricular activities, future expectations, self-image, and work orientation. These between-sex differences are important because other data-based studies have demonstrated differences between boys and girls, as, for example, lower self-image in girls (Petersen, Offer, and Kaplan 1979). The Offer Self-Image Questionnaire for Adolescents (Offer and Howard 1972), an instrument used in previous studies, was also used in the present one, and a detailed analysis of between-sex differences, as well as correlations of self-image with such things as level of family competence, will be detailed in a future work.

Caution should be used to avoid generalizing too broadly from the findings of this study for several reasons. One is that the youngsters in the two samples were preselected for superior psychologic functioning. The findings therefore do not answer the question of how similar (or dissimilar) poor, black and wealthier, white adolescents would be if adolescents with broader ranges of psychological functioning were compared. In addition, the sample sizes in both groups of the present comparison are not large enough to enable one to draw definitive conclusions, and there was no control group. The findings of this study, therefore, although reaching statistical significance, need to be replicated, using samples of larger size with controls. Despite these caveats, the findings of this preliminary study suggest that, at a time when there is increasing stress on the family and when more and more children are being raised in fragmented families, even under far from optimal social conditions, living in an intact family that functions well facilitates highly adaptive levels of functioning in adolescent family members.

Summary

In this report two groups of adolescents have been compared and contrasted—black adolescents from working-class families and white adolescents from middle- and upper-middle-class families. The comparisons were based on detailed content analyses of intensive interviews. Although from very different neighborhoods, levels of family income, and life opportunities, the adolescents in these two groups shared an important asset. They were from families determined by rigorous research methodology to be functioning at the more competent end of the continuum of family competence. A preliminary hypothesis that ethnic and socioeconomic forces would cause these two groups of adolescents to be very dissimilar was incorrect. The similarities were, in fact, striking. This important research finding underscores the power of the family as the crucible of human development.

NOTES

We wish to acknowledge the assistance of F. David Barnhart, M.A., and Joseph T. Gossett, Ph.D., in the preparation of this manuscript. We also wish to thank Susan B. Looney for her editorial review.

1. Family competence is defined as the capacity to produce autonomous children and provide emotional support for the parents.

2. John T. Gossett, Ph.D., Jerry M. Lewis, M.D., and John G. Looney, M.D.

3. In the second study, the adolescents also completed the Offer Self-Image Questionnaire for Adolescents, and the results correlated significantly with the interview ratings ($r = .58, P < .01$).

4. The Hollingshead "Four-Factor Index of Social Position" was used to check the assumption that these families fell toward the lower end of the continuum of social status within the greater community. The mean index score for the group was 4.5. In the United States, the primary wage earner from families at this level would be involved in activities ranging from menial service and unskilled labor through semiskilled labor and machine operation.

5. In contrast, black adolescents who rated at less than average levels of adaptation came from families with an average family competence rating of 6.2 ($P < .01$).

REFERENCES

Blos, P. *On Adolescence*. 1962. New York: Free Press.

Blotcky, M. J., and Looney, J. G. 1980. Normal female and male adolescent psychological development: an overview of theory and research. *Adolescent Psychiatry* 8:184–199.

Dallas Morning News. 1981. March 26.

Douvan, E., and Adelson, J. 1966. *The Adolescent Experience*. New York: Wiley.

Erikson, E. 1956. The program of ego identity. *Journal of the American Psychoanalytic Association* 4:56–121.

Freud, A. Adolescence. 1958. *The Psychoanalytic Study of the Child* 13:255–278.

Hall, G. S. 1904. *Adolescence: Its Psychology and Its Relations to Physiology, Anthropology, Sociobiology, Sex, Crime, Religion and Education*. Vols. 1, 2. New York: Appleton-Century-Crofts.

Josselyn, I. 1954. The ego in adolescence. *American Journal of Orthopsychiatry* 24:223–237.

Lewis, J. M.; Beavers, W. R.; Gossett, J. T.; and Phillips, V. A. 1976. *No Single Thread: Psychological Health in Family Systems.* New York: Brunner/Mazel.

Lindemann, E. 1964. Adolescent behavior as a community concern. *American Journal of Psychotherapy* 18:204–417.

Looney, J. G., and Gunderson, E. K. E. 1978. Transient situation disorders: a longitudinal study in young men. *American Journal of Psychiatry* 135:660–663.

Masterson, J. 1967. *The Psychiatric Dilemma of Adolescence.* Boston: Little, Brown.

Mead, M. 1928. *Coming of Age in Samoa.* New York: Morrow.

Mead, M. 1930. Adolescence in primitive and modern society. In F. V. Calverton and S. D. Schmalhausen, eds. *The New Generation: A Symposium.* New York: Macauley.

Offer, D. 1969. *The Psychological World of the Teenager.* New York: Basic.

Offer, D., and Howard, K. I. 1972. "The Offer Self-Image Questionnaire for Adolescents." *Archives of General Psychiatry* 27:529–537.

Oldham, D. G. 1978. Adolescent turmoil: a myth revisited. *Journal of Continuing Education in Psychiatry* 39:23–32.

Petersen, A. C.; Offer, D.; and Kaplan, E. 1979. Self image of rural adolescent girls. In M. Sugar, ed. *Female Adolescent Development.* New York: Brunner/Mazel.

Spiegel, L. 1961. Identity and adolescence. In S. Lorand and H. I. Schneer, eds. *Adolescents: Psychoanalytic Approach to Problems and Therapy.* New York: Hoeber.

Vaillant, G. E. 1977. *Adaptation to Life.* Boston: Little, Brown.

Weiner, I., and Del Gaudio, A. 1976. Psychopathology in adolescence. *Archives of General Psychiatry* 33:187–193.

7   THE FAIRY TALE AS PARADIGM OF THE SEPARATION-INDIVIDUATION CRISIS: IMPLICATIONS FOR TREATMENT OF THE BORDERLINE ADOLESCENT

LAURIE M. BRANDT

Fairy tales offer vital solutions for mastering life, growth, and development. The following is an exploration of the fairy tale as paradigm of the separation-individuation crisis of early childhood, with particular reference to its implications for work with borderline patients. That fairy tales can serve important ego integrative functions in the normal development of the child has been described by Bettelheim (1976) and Schwartz (1956). Since the borderline syndrome is thought to represent a developmental failure during the separation-individuation phase, this chapter explores the function of fairy tales for normal children, the particular use made of them by the borderline, and the relation of the two, with possible implications for treatment. The theoretical material will be highlighted by the case of a borderline adolescent who made use of two "brother-sister" tales to soothe and integrate herself when anxious. The patient's pleasure and investment in these specific fairy tales at this time in her life raises questions about the purposes they might be serving for her in the context of therapeutic and extratherapeutic events.

The Case of Clare

Clare is a twenty-one-year-old single white female who began psychotherapy following graduation from college and a move to a new city in July 1979. She came to therapy reporting severe "anxiety attacks" with "fear of the unknown," beginning at age fifteen, upon first leaving home for boarding school. At these times, the patient soothes herself by "going to bed and reading a fairy tale." Favorite among these are Hans Christian Andersen's "The Snow Queen" (1930) and C. S. Lewis's *The Lion, the Witch, and the Wardrobe* (1950), in which, she says, "Good against evil, and good triumphs—very idealistic and happy."

Clare is one of four siblings from a wealthy family. A fifth sibling, a brother three years her senior, died of leukemia at age twenty-two, following an eighteen-month illness. Her present family members are: a fifty-eight-year-old father, a businessman who is quite well respected in the community but described as "childish, emotional and seductive" at home; a fifty-five-year-old mother, a housewife who does volunteer work and is described as "all-knowing, all-calm" but somewhat cold, unemotional, and unavailable; a sister, age twenty-eight, a student; a brother, age twenty-seven, a recovering alcoholic and the only family member to move to a different part of the country; and a sister, age sixteen, currently attending boarding school. Family relations are described as quite enmeshed, particularly since the brother's death, with everybody "sticking together like glue." There is evidence that separations from the family were difficult for Clare even before her brother's death. She describes herself as "a little baby spider plant," presenting the illusion of independence while always connected to her parents. Indicative of this difficulty is her statement that "traveling alone would be like taking cyanide."

Although Clare has revealed little about her early childhood, she described age six as her first time of crisis, marking the occasion of three important losses. These were the death of paternal grandmother; beginning school; and, perhaps most important, the experienced loss of her mother through the birth of her younger sister. Clare describes this sibling as mother's favorite, but maintains her own position of "baby of the family" through continuing temper tantrums.

It seems that Clare was able to function fairly well through her latency years, until reaching puberty at age twelve. While it is unclear what observable shifts took place at this time, Clare feels that she is "developmentally arrested" at age twelve—as, she says, is her father, who experienced a similar "insular, protected" upbringing. She describes those traits of twelve-year-old girls with which she most identifies as "bitchy, fighting, struggling with blossoming woman-hood."

The next time of major difficulty for Clare was at age fifteen when she first left home for boarding school. It was here that she first experienced an "anxiety attack," described as follows:

> Sometimes when I least expect it, sometimes very predictably, I become anxious, a bottomless fear overwhelms me. I guess I am afraid of being afraid. It's a fear of myself, I think. I really don't know. It has been six years since this all began. It is by no means a constant problem. But knowing that this feeling of dread can return nags at me. I am always on guard.

Behavior difficulties accompanied her anxiety, and Clare was expelled from school at the end of this year. She was then sent to a second boarding school, somewhat closer to home, where she managed to complete the last two years of high school, still suffering intermittent anxiety.

The next period of major difficulty for Clare was her brother's illness, and eventual death, while she was at college in another state. She refers to this brother as her "soul mate" and regrets that she never told him she loved him. She currently becomes panic-stricken when she finds herself unable to remember what he looked like and has begun to write down memories about him for fear that she will forget these as well. Lately Clare has revealed that at times she does not believe that her brother is actually dead, since she never saw his body. It seems significant that Clare was never able to cry over her brother's death prior to therapy but has done so in therapy in a controlled fashion, saying "I never cry for more than ten minutes. I'm afraid I'll lose control if I do."

Shortly after her brother's death, Clare became involved with a male student at school. This was described as a "strong mutual dependency" which she eventually terminated because she felt herself to be "merging" with him. Following this, she allowed herself to enter into no intimate relationships for over a year, when she became involved with a man who was leaving town in three months and thus was "safe."

Clare referred herself to outpatient psychotherapy following another major shift in her life, graduation from college and a move to a new city. In examining her own historical points of emphasis, it seems clear that, although this girl has managed to function fairly well, times of separation, loss, and change were most difficult for her. These were death of grandmother; beginning school; birth of her younger sister when Clare was age six; puberty at age twelve; beginning boarding school at age fifteen; death of her brother when she was nineteen; graduation from college; and relocation at age twenty-one. Similar difficulties were echoed in the course of therapy when she described herself as "falling apart" during the therapist's vacation, or when she had difficulty maintaining an evocative image of the therapist between appointments.

Early in the course of treatment, it became clear that, despite this patient's reasonably high level of functioning, she did seem to have an essentially borderline personality organization. This was supported by her affective lability, pervasive anxiety, loose boundaries (mixing pronouns between herself and the therapist), difficulty with evocative imagery (in regard to her brother and therapist), extreme alienation from her own motivational system, identity diffusion ("I'm saying all these things that don't sound like they're me at all"), and a tendency to split.

Splitting, as Clare uses it, involves an inability to integrate disparate feelings, or rather, an inability to experience herself as a continuous person when she experiences disparate feelings. Further, she tends to see objects as "all good" or "all bad," as in her description of her mother as "all-knowing" and of her father as a "jerk." These perceptions seem largely to be linked to her need states and seem to stem from a relative failure in achieving object constancy. Consistent with this notion is her inability with regard to evocative imagery (Mahler 1968, 1975).

Clare's personal manner of consoling herself following losses and of controlling overwhelming anxiety has been to "get into bed and read a fairy tale." While these attempts were ultimately unsuccessful in terms of permanently warding off or understanding her anxiety, they do seem to offer an invaluable opportunity to better understand the developmental tasks of early childhood, the developmental failures of the borderline, and the ego integrative tasks for psychotherapeutic work with such patients. In the following, I will explore the fairy tale, particularly the "sister-brother" tales such as "The Snow Queen" (Andersen 1930) and *The Lion, the Witch, and the Wardrobe* (Lewis 1950); their echoing and attempted resolution of the splitting phenomenon;

the specific use made of them by Clare; and implications for psycho-therapy with borderline adolescents and young adults.

The Fairy Tale: Its Uses in Development

Fairy tales "represent in imaginative form what the process of healthy human development consists of, and . . . make such development attractive for the child to engage in" (Bettelheim 1976, p. 12). Their essential nature is didactic or instructional, with the conscious or unconscious intent of working through developmental problems. They echo the struggles of development with a veneer of fantasy that allows the child to find meaning in them without being overwhelmed; and they provide models for mastery of both the inner problems of growth and development and the external world of human relations.

One use of the fairy tale is the support of ego growth and the control of instinctual pressures through the ego and superego development that it fosters. With its balance between primary and secondary processes, it serves to promote ego integration while allowing for the appropriate satisfaction of id wishes as well.

Fairy tales, particularly enduring ones, offer models for, and solutions to, the child's dilemmas at many levels of development. Which tale is most meaningful to a child depends on both his developmental stage and his current problems. One of the most common themes of the fairy tale is separation from home and family, or from rightful heritage, or by death. It seems no accident that the fairy tale is commonly read at bedtime, when fear of relinquishing ego controls and separation anxiety are at their peak. It is in this light that the story's typically "happy ending" seems especially important. By experiencing the triumphs of good over evil and reunion following separation prior to falling asleep, one is able to deny momentarily the power of the primary process and relinquish controls sufficiently to separate and go to sleep. This may also explain in part the appeal and usefulness of the fairy tale for the borderline adolescent.

While the fairy tale reflects the many struggles of childhood and the developing ego, perhaps most crucial in these stories is their wide-spread use of splitting. The figures in fairy tales are not ambivalent, not good and bad at the same moment, but clearly divided into all-good and all-bad objects. This echoes the young child's ego structure and serves the same purpose for him: it keeps the good object uncontaminated by the bad; and it allows expression of aggression at the bad object without fear of injuring the good.

But the fairy tale goes beyond a portrayal of splitting; it offers a model for ego and object integration as well. Not only does good triumph over evil, but an integration of disparate elements often takes place in the resolution of a happy, though ordinary, existence. Such is the case in what may be referred to as the "sister-brother" stories, in which two siblings, usually male and female, represent opposite and often conflicting elements to be integrated in the course of human development. In many of these stories (e.g., the Grimms' "Brother and Sister" [1944]), siblings represent id versus primitive ego and superego, with integration of these disparate elements by the story's end through ego growth and development. In other brother and sister stories (e.g., "The Snow Queen" [Andersen 1930] and *The Lion, the Witch, and the Wardrobe* [Lewis 1950]), while the split is still between instinctual gratification and the ability to control and delay, the brother and sister come for a time to themselves represent good and evil, which are then reunited and integrated in the end.

The Lion, the Witch, and the Wardrobe (Lewis 1950) will now be reviewed in an attempt to sort out some of its meanings and importance for the young child in normal development, for Clare, and perhaps for the borderline adolescent in general. This has been chosen over the similar "The Snow Queen" (Andersen 1930) because of its greater richness and embellishment of an essentially identical story.

The story begins with four children being separated from their parents and sent to a large house in the English countryside to protect them from wartime air raids in London. During a game of hide-and-seek, the youngest child, six-year-old Lucy, enters into the magical kingdom of Narnia through a wardrobe full of coats. The next to enter is Edmund, the youngest boy, who becomes seduced by the evil White Witch who provides him with instinctual gratification by feeding him an irresistible Turkish delight. The older children, also a girl and a boy, enter Narnia as well, but for a time the two youngest come to be the human embodiments of good and evil, to be separated and then reunited as the story evolves.

It should be noted that this was the precise composition of Clare's own family, with her being the youngest until the birth of her sister when she was six, and with her now deceased brother preceding her in birth order. The notion of four children being left to their own resources in the large house, without benefit of adult supervision or caretaking, is consistent with Clare's own history, particularly at age six, when her mother was involved with her pregnancy and then with the care of her youngest daughter. It seems likely that the White Witch, malevolent and cold, may have represented for Clare her own "bad mother," whose withdrawal was particularly painful at this time and whose coldness she often refers to even now.

The broader theme of the tale involves a conflict between the evil White Witch (parallel to the Snow Queen) and the all-good lion Aslan, with Aslan not taking power himself upon his victory but giving the four children the joint reign over Narnia. While good does triumph over evil, the resolution was not to retain the all-good object but to move toward greater integration in the form of the generally good, but imperfect, children. Even Aslan himself represents a beginning integration between disparate elements (Lewis 1950, p. 123):

People who have not been in Narnia sometimes think that a thing cannot be good and terrible at the same time. If the children had ever thought so, they were cured of it now. For when they tried to look at Aslan's face they just caught a glimpse of the golden mane and the great, royal, solemn, overwhelming eyes, and then they found they couldn't look at him and went all trembling.

While these stories are used in general by young children in an attempt to achieve greater integration and solutions to the many struggles of growing up, it seems likely that they may serve parallel purposes later in life when similar crises are activated. Cath and Cath (1978, p. 622) support this view in speaking of the parent who, in reading the fairy tale to his child, has "another opportunity to rework some of [his] own childhood conflicts related to age-specific tasks at hand." Similarly, it does not seem surprising for a borderline adolescent to make use of the fairy tale in such a fashion. This particular choice of tale, in fact, seems the ideal vehicle for dealing with the reactivation of the separation-individuation struggle in adolescence and with the borderline's accompanying use of splitting.

Aspects of the Therapy

I will now examine two specific instances in the treatment of Clare where her reference to and use of fairy tales or derivatives from them were most striking. The first selections are from session 1 when initial references to *The Lion, the Witch, and the Wardrobe* (Lewis 1950) were made. The second came five months later, in the seventeenth session of her psychotherapy, when certain therapeutic and extra-therapeutic events seem to have reactivated separation-individuation issues for her.

SESSION 1

Clare entered this first session with intense anxiety, initially speaking about the various changes in her life that she had just experienced: graduation from college; move to a new city; beginning a new job; and beginning therapy. This led her to a discussion of the "anxiety attacks" that she had been experiencing since high school, the recurrence of which she was particularly fearful about at this time.

> PATIENT: See I've gotten so good at controlling it that I can stop it before it starts . . . by going to be by myself and totally turn . . . like avoid my mind. I go read a book or just turn it off sort of.

This led her to a more detailed description of the physical symptomatology of her anxiety, of the early history of these attacks, and of her uncertainty about the future. Clare then expressed the need to separate or "box off" the different aspects of her life, especially events from feelings, in a manner that seemed to defy integration or any experience of herself as a continuous person over time or across relationships.

> THERAPIST: They're somehow easier to think about when you box them off like that?
> PATIENT: Um-hum. When I can just like put them in a category. Problem: family. Problem: my brother's death. Problem: my future. It is because then I can say, enough, okay, away.
> THERAPIST: Kind of like how you, when you're feeling anxious . . . read a book to get things out of your mind.
> PATIENT: Um-hum. . . . A lot of times the kind of book I read—I have a bookcase by my bed, and the books in it—95 percent of them are fairy-tale books, and if I'm all uptight I'll pull out, you know, Hans Christian Andersen, a fairy tale, or I'll pull out an anthology of short stories, and it's something that's so remote from reality. Just, it gets me through the night. . . .

THERAPIST: What's your favorite fairy tale?

PATIENT: What's my favorite fairy tale? Oh, I like a lot of them. Um . . . I guess—I love "The Snow Queen." I think that's my favorite one.

THERAPIST: What do you like about it?

PATIENT: . . . It's like *The Lion, the Witch, and the Wardrobe* is a lot—it's almost the same story I would think. It's kind of a good story—good against evil, and good triumphs. Very idealistic and happy. . . .

Both Clare's anxiety at this time and her reference to these fairy tales seem closely linked to the major life changes, including beginning therapy, that she was experiencing. Just as earlier changes and separations had highlighted faulty developmental processes and made evident borderline pathology in this girl, the many shifts occurring at this time in her life seem to have challenged again Clare's limited capacity for individuation. Most striking here are her clear lack of object constancy and continuity across time and space, as evidenced by her need to categorize and isolate affect. This lack of object constancy, which became increasingly obvious in the following sessions, is typified in Clare by a virtual inability to evoke mental images of lost objects, most evident in relation to her dead brother and the therapist. Just as Clare's inability to evoke a stable mental image of her brother had prevented her from being soothed by such an image and from resolving painful feelings of loss sufficiently to truly mourn or to form new object relations, similarly, separations from the therapist were met with an inability to evoke her image or to gain comfort and sustenance from it. While this failure was most striking following more extended absences, such as vacations, at times Clare also had difficulty between appointments and found it necessary to supplement hours by frequent telephone contact. Significantly, this patient had particular inability to evoke a stable mental image of the therapist following what was experienced as an empathic break. While the child who has successfully completed early separation-individuation and achieved object constancy is able to maintain object relatedness irrespective of frustration or satisfaction, and thus to tolerate separations from the mother, Clare's marked loss of the object following frustration highlights her borderline personality organization and early developmental fixation.

Her references to fairy tales and to these particular fairy tales at this time—*The Lion, the Witch, and the Wardrobe*—quite clearly address issues of separation. These are the children's separation from their parents by the war, followed by the split between Lucy and Edmund, and emphasized at various points in the story by both physical separations and the fear of loss by death, and of reunion or integration. One might hypothesize that the power to soothe that this story holds for Clare lies both in its echoing of her predicament and the normalizing sense of "not being alone" that this communicates and, perhaps more important, in its attempt to resolve the splits and to integrate what Clare refers to as the "idealistic and happy" ending. It seems quite likely that this patient makes use of the fairy tale in much the same way as the small child: to highlight significant developmental issues in a symbolic, nonthreatening form and to suggest and make attractive growth and integration.

The next interchange, somewhat later in therapy, occurred following what the patient experienced as an empathic break which forced acknowledgment of her own separateness and refers to a portion of the story more specifically tied to the struggle for integration.

SESSION 17

The stimulus for this session seemed to arise three and one-half weeks previously, in the fourteenth session of her therapy. Up to this point, Clare had established a rather idealized view of the therapist as an all-bountiful caretaker and nurturer. In this session, however, the therapist brought to her attention the fact that she had not paid for several of her therapy hours. This confrontation seems to have been experienced by the patient in two ways. First, it was felt as an attack, an empathic rupture which forced her to look at her own separateness and at the professional nature of the therapeutic relationship. Second, this interchange seems to have exposed the demanding and manipulative Clare who does not meet her responsibilities and wants to receive without giving, a self-image quite intolerable to her. Immediately following this, she expressed thoughts about discontinuing therapy and then devalued the therapist, saying that her interpretations captured "the skeleton [of Clare], but not the meat" and made the therapist sound "cold and calculating." This was an apparent attempt to disown and split off the intolerable image of herself as greedy or demanding and to project it onto the therapist.

That this girl should so easily alternate between an idealized and a devalued view of the therapist seems again related to her essential failure to achieve object constancy. Just as the young child uses splitting both to prevent diffusion of anxiety within the ego and to protect positive introjects and identifications, Clare continues to use this mechanism in her effort to keep both the responsible, satiable Clare separate from the manipulative, greedy Clare and the good mother-therapist separate from the bad mother-therapist.

In the following session (15), Clare continually questioned the therapist's ability to care for and be a "good mother" to her. This contrasted with her previous idealization and apparently was a direct reaction to her disappointment of the previous hour. She noticed a space heater in the office and became terrified that the therapist would not be able to provide enough warmth for her; no longer was Clare "cold and calculating," it was now the therapist as receptacle for her projections who was cold. The major part of the session, however, dealt with her two female managers at work, whom she had, in previous sessions, typically polarized with positive and negative affect. In contrast to earlier hours, however, Clare seemed, in this discussion, to make beginning attempts at integration. Previously polarization had been complete, but now she seemed to move closer to integration in that she included both positive and negative elements in one session and was for moments able to see the managers as complex rather than unidimensional figures.

Clare canceled the next session and came thirty-five minutes late for the rescheduled hour. The relationship between this avoidance of the therapist and the experienced rupture of session 14 seemed clear in her complaints about a veterinarian's bill and the "brickfaced woman" who claimed to understand, and perhaps did, but still made her pay. She then reported extreme agitation on several nights, insomnia, and turning to her typical method of soothing with bedtime reading of fairy tales.

These events seem to be the background for session 17 in which Clare alludes in derivative to Aslan, the powerful, yet just, lion of the Narnia stories, in what seems to be a beginning attempt to integrate disparate affects and attributes both in others and in herself. In addition to the above-mentioned therapeutic events, Clare had ambivalently resigned from her job during the week preceding this hour. Just before the interchange to be related, she found herself fluctuating between feelings of helplessness and feelings of grandiosity.

THERAPIST: You can do anything, and you're relatively free, but you don't sound very pleased about that.

PATIENT: I am, but I don't know what that means. . . . I don't know what that will mean for me. What act . . . how I will use that. So that I'm not unhappy about it, but I'm just kinda' like a little puzzled. That's no news. . . .

THERAPIST: What are your limitations?

PATIENT: Oh, well, there are obvious monetary limitations. I can't go to Russia.

THERAPIST: To Russia?

PATIENT: I don't know . . . anyplace. I can't go to the Gold Coast of Africa. I'd love to go there. You know the lions play on the beach on the Gold Coast of Africa. Wouldn't that be great to see? . . . [This is an allusion to Aslan in derivative form. It is consistent with other indirect fairy tale references throughout Clare's psychotherapy. The specific image of the lion "on the beach on the Gold Coast of Africa" is most likely a condensation of a number of different portrayals of Aslan—on the "Lone Islands"; in the "Extreme East"; in "Aslan's Country" at the "Far end of the world"—found in subsequent volumes of Lewis's *Chronicles of Narnia*].

THERAPIST: What's so nice for you about the lions playing on the beach?

PATIENT: Um, it's just such an incongruent image to me. I mean, lions, I picture them sitting on a hot plain, under a shady tree, just hanging out panting or something. But to see them, to—in my mind I see them—playing on white sand, blue sky, just water everywhere, is just so different. The two images are totally, completely different to me, and I would just love to see it.

THERAPIST: Do they seem ferocious in that image?

PATIENT: No, they're not. The lions are almost playful. I don't know. It would be interesting. . . .

THERAPIST: And it's the two images, or the ferocious beasts being playful . . . what's so . . . you look very pleased.

PATIENT: I don't know. It just seems like a neat thing. I don't know. I just thought it would be fun to see. It's like something out of another world that doesn't fit with . . . it doesn't really fit with my image of what lions should do or something. So it's out of the ordinary. So it's . . . appealing. It's, um, I don't know, it's like my old boyfriend Jim—he's writing a book. That's about as incongruent as you could get.

THERAPIST: How's that?

PATIENT: I love the idea of it. I think it's great. Because, um, well, since he's been 17, he's been traveling pretty much. . . . He's been living in the Middle East pretty consistently for a long time, and he has a really hard time speaking English. . . . He'll not hear English for such a long period of time that he's really funny. . . . It's really funny cause he gets his grammar all mixed up, and, um, he took an English course, and he just had the hardest time. . . . It was awful, and he just suffered over these papers, and now he's writing a book, and that's just . . . it's great, but it's totally, it's just like, I can't wait to see it cause it's so out of the ordinary.

THERAPIST: So the ferocious beasts are playful; the guy who can't speak English is writing a book. So it looks like anything's possible.

PATIENT: Uh-huh. Yeah. Yeah. The things in life to me that are most precious and special, as I look back, are the things that I did that I never thought I had it in me type things.

THERAPIST: Like what?

PATIENT: Like, uh, Oh God, climbing a water tower that's like sixty feet high . . . at five o'clock in the morning to watch the sun rise. Or . . . climbing Mt. Mansfield. Climbing is something that I never think I have in me until I do it. Climbing Mt. Mansfield, the hardest trail on the mountain.

This hour illustrates Clare's typical use of splitting and her attempts to integrate—the pathology and the growth at once. While it does seem that she may well be attempting to split off and deny the ferocity of the lions by making them playful and peaceful, which parallels her typically disowning her own aggression in the therapy, this association seems to be clearly an attempt at integration in her repeated references to the "incongruity." While this girl's earlier statements had been clear-cut, one-sided references without any examination of incongruity or sense that it could be otherwise, the work of therapy had been a continual pointing out of contradictions and attempts to make real for her her own continuity across time, relationships, and disparate affects. While removing the aggression is perhaps a form of splitting, and indeed, her "loving" such incongruity is an illustration of her reluctance to renounce such primitive mechanisms, her current capacity to note and appreciate that this is an incongruity must be considered an important step toward greater integration.

Reference to the boyfriend seems a further step in this direction in that it is less removed from human experience. Just as incongruent to Clare as "lions playing on the beach" is the idea of this young man who had had trouble speaking but is now writing a book. Predominant in this vignette is an idea of struggle preceding accomplishment. Similarly, Clare appears to have a sense that in the therapy one has to experience a painful uncovering and struggle before accomplishment. While this type of thinking is still a step away from the notion of cause and effect—struggle merely precedes accomplishment but does not yet lead to it—it does seem to be a precursor to an acquisition of cause-and-effect thinking, with the ego growth and integration implicit in this.

The grandiose "I can do anything" notion expressed at the end of session 17 can be considered both in terms of its elements of denial and those of integration, its defensive and its adaptive functions. While, on the one hand, Clare here denies and disowns her own sense of entrapment and helplessness by means of her grandiosity, she also vaguely begins to become aware of her own capacities, of the possibility of working toward a goal, and of gratification through accomplishment.

The transcripts of this session and of the three previous hours, then, indicate that the following sequence occurred:

1. The therapist's reference to money was experienced as a rejection, creating separate boundaries for both, and as an empathic break leading to:

2. Forced awareness of her separateness from the therapist and the accompanying separation anxiety and anxiety about "badness" in herself to explain the rejection;

3. Splitting of the therapist into the "good" and "bad" mothers;

4. Increased anxiety and attempts to soothe/reintegrate herself by bedtime reading;

5. Splitting shifted to in an attempt to integrate by allowing both positive and negative elements in a single hour (female managers); and in her beginning queries about incongruities in others (lions, boyfriend) and in herself (helplessness/grandiosity); and in the emergence of cause and effect in session 17.

This session points clearly to the role that the Narnia story has for this girl, not only as an object of comfort or normalizing but as a vehicle toward integration of disparate elements in her ongoing struggles with separation-individuation. It also points to the more subtle, implicit use that one can make of appropriate fairy-tale material and to the recurrent valence of certain stories for individuals that is based on the specific developmental issues that they address.

Implications

If we look at borderline pathology as representing a developmental arrest during the rapprochement subphase of early separation-individuation, then treatment of such patients must consist of successful passage through this subphase with the ego development and integration that this would entail. Therapy with these patients must work toward the development of autonomous ego functioning, the strengthening of ego controls over instinctual impulses, and the maturation of the defensive and adaptive functions of the ego.

With this view in mind, let us turn to our understanding of the fairy tale in search of treatment implications. The most obvious possibility would involve direct use of the fairy tale in treatment. This approach is most feasible when the material is brought spontaneously by the patient, as in the case of Clare, and might involve direct interpretation of the fairy-tale symbolism or direct reference to previously mentioned fairy-tale material, much as one might refer to life events or dreams at appropriate times in the therapy. A second, and perhaps more valuable, use of the fairy tale is as a vehicle for understanding the transference. Just as the fairy-tale figures are split into those who are good and bad, in reflection of the young child's primitive ego functioning, the borderline patient, in the context of the transference, may see the therapist at different times as purely good or bad or, more correctly, as embodying either good or bad part-objects. The specific fairy-tale reference, then, may help the therapist to understand the transference paradigm. Similarly, one must consider the role of countertransference in evoking fairy-tale references. The assault on our own boundaries by the patient's unipolar projections may be so powerful and manipulative as to lead us either to fulfill her projections and be either the "fairy godmother" or the "witch" or to attempt to rid ourselves of the projections in a manner that abandons objectivity.

The fairy tale, then, may be used directly in the psychotherapy of borderline patients as an echoing of their developmental struggles subject to interpretation, as a window into the transference phenomenon, or as a warning of insidious countertransference. The most important use of the fairy tale, however, seems not in its direct use at all but in its use as a model.

The fairy tale, for some patients, can serve as paradigm for the ego integrative work of psychotherapy with borderline patients. It begins where the primitive ego is and holds out the promise of growth through integration; it repeats its message over and over again in different ways and from different perspectives so that it is gradually introjected without being overwhelming; it provides structure and emphasizes the importance of caring human relationships while at the same time promoting autonomy and individuation. In other words, while the fairy tale may not be an explicit element in psychotherapy with most patients, it does seem to offer a model for work with all patients who have experienced developmental failure or ego deficits. As the young child makes use of the fairy tale both to echo his developmental struggles and to resolve them, and as Clare creatively attempts to do the same in her effort to resolve conflicts and integrate disparate elements never coalesced in childhood, so we as therapists need to address and aid the integrative tasks never completed in the borderline's early development.

Summary

This chapter is an attempt to offer a model for therapeutic work with borderline patients that is based on the structure and content of the fairy tale. It views the fairy tale as both descriptive in its echoing of developmental struggles of childhood and integrative in providing a model for resolution of these conflicts. Clare's use of the fairy tale offers confirmation of theoretical notions which place the etiology of borderline pathology in early developmental failures and a clue to the therapeutic work with borderline patients. While the childhood route of the fairy tale may no longer be available to most, its subtle mirroring of the separation-individuation crisis and gradual, growthful steps toward integration of both the external and the internal worlds offer an exquisite model for the work of psychotherapy.

"Once a king in Narnia, always a king in Narnia.

But don't go trying to use the same route twice. . ." (Lewis 1950, p. 186).

REFERENCES

Andersen, H. C. 1930. *Favourite Tales of Hans Andersen*. Translated by M. R. James. London: Faber & Faber, 1978.

Bettelheim, B. 1976. *The Uses of Enchantment: The Meaning and Importance of Fairy Tales*. New York: Knopf.

Cath, S. H., and Cath, C. 1978. On the other side of Oz: psychoanalytic aspects of fairy tales. *Psychoanalytic Study of the Child* 33:621–640.

Grimm, Brothers. 1944 Brother and sister. *Complete Grimm's Fairy Tales*. New York: Pantheon.

Lewis, C. S. 1950. *The Chronicles of Narnia*. Vol. 1, *The Lion, the Witch, and the Wardrobe*. New York: Collier, 1978.

Mahler, M. 1968. *On Human Symbiosis and the Vicissitudes of Individuation*. New York: International Universities Press.

Mahler, M. 1975. *The Psychological Birth of the Human Infant*. New York: Basic.

Schwartz, E. K. 1956. A psychoanalytic study of the fairy tale. *American Journal of Psychotherapy* 10:740–762.

91

8 THE DIARY AS A TRANSITIONAL OBJECT IN FEMALE ADOLESCENT DEVELOPMENT

DEBORAH ANNE SOSIN

> 20 June 1942
> I haven't written for a few days, because I wanted first
> of all to think about my diary. It's an odd idea for
> someone like me to keep a diary; not only because it
> seems to me that neither I—nor for that matter anyone
> else—will be interested in the unbosomings of a
> thirteen-year-old schoolgirl. Still, what does that mat-
> ter? I want to write, but more than that, I want to bring
> out all kinds of things that lie buried deep in my heart.
> [ANNE FRANK]

Each night, thousands of young women throughout the world turn to their diaries to vent feelings, record daily activities, and write about their fears and fantasies. Teenage diaries afford an evocative glimpse into the adolescent mind. Themes of love, friendship, disillusionment, selfhood, and loss dominate the pages written by these expressive young women. The act of writing, however, is not merely an intellectual activity; there is an emotional component and developmental function to the diary-diarist relationship. A girl may form an intense attachment to her diary—carrying it from place to place, fearing its discovery, and cherishing the intimacy it provides.

In this chapter, I review aspects of adolescent diary writing relevant to the understanding of the diary-diarist relationship. Materials gathered from retrospective interviews and verbatim diary excerpts illustrate the diary's function as a transitional object in female adolescent development.

Review of the Literature

The psychological literature gives scant attention to the phenomenon of adolescent diary writing. When mentioned, diary writing is primarily described as a female activity which provides an outlet for a girl's thoughts and feelings. With few exceptions, noted below, the literature overlooks the relational and developmental functions of a diary.

The primary developmental task of adolescence is to relinquish the emotional ties of the past and create new ones (Deutsch 1944). Blos (1967) labeled this transitional period the "second individuation process," a time when earlier infantile issues of separation and individuation are revived and condensed. In an effort to substitute for the exclusive tie to the parent, adolescents may form intensified relationships to abstractions such as ideas, nature, or religion, or to inanimate objects such as cars, drugs, or books (Group for the Advancement of Psychiatry 1968). The teenage diary becomes a safe, private, all-accepting partner—a transitional object—which facilitates the passage into adulthood.

Adolescent Diary Writing

In 1919, *A Young Girl's Diary* (Hug-Hellmuth) was published anonymously with a preface written by Freud. The diary attracted considerable interest in the Viennese psychoanalytic community for its frank, uncensored portrait of adolescent development. Later, Bernfeld (1927) examined the content of girls' diaries and concluded that adolescent diaries have minimal usefulness for therapists. He believed they represented only the conscious manifestation of the diarist's feelings and revealed little unconscious material. Bernfeld's content-focused approach may have precluded exploration of the relational and developmental functions of a diary.

Blos (1962) mentioned the diary's use as an object and postulated several normal functions of diaries, including trying out new role identifications, releasing tensions that might lead to premature heterosexual acting out, and aiding the ego in its task of synthesis and mastery.

As an outgrowth of what Elkind (1971) called "adolescent egocentrism," the diarist creates an "imaginary audience" in her diary, in which aspects of her self are reflected back to her. In this sense, the diary's mirroring function is similar to the mother's mirroring function in early childhood as described by Kohut (1971) and contributes to the development of normal narcissism. Scarlett (1971) examined the content of Anne Frank's diary and concluded that the diary can be useful as evidence of adolescent developmental processes.

Baruch's (1968→1969) discussion of Anne Frank's diary went beyond a content analysis. She acknowledged the diary's function as an object during the transitional phase of adolescence:

> In a state of object hunger, taking the self as a love object can mitigate emptiness and protect against a severe sense of inadequacy. Cathexes of the sense organs and a heightened ego feeling contribute to the inner awareness and increased activity. Anne's diary permits the expression of such feelings and also stands as proof that she possesses a treasure of important thoughts and secrets. [P. 430]

Baruch acknowledged the importance of Anne's diary as a passive container for her emotions. However, she overlooked the adaptive, interactive process that takes place between the girl and her diary in the service of differentiation.

There is consensus in the available literature that diary writing is a far more common activity for girls than for boys. Blos (1962) suggested that diary writing has connotations of femininity and passivity. He stated that boys in this society tend to seek aggressive, extroverted activities, while girls may be more compelled by the emotional self-absorption implicit in diary keeping. In a less judgmental way, Gilligan (1982) proposed that girls may be drawn toward activities with a strong relational component, whereas boys may develop values that are predominantly based on logic and rationality (Kohlberg 1981). As assignment of "sex-appropriate" activities changes in modern society, girls *and* boys may learn to engage comfortably in both "passive" and "active" ventures of their choosing.

This chapter builds on the work of the above-mentioned authors and examines the phase-appropriate use of the diary as a transitional object.

Transitional Objects

The concept of the transitional object was first developed by Winnicott in his landmark paper of 1953. He used the term to describe those objects and activities which serve as "substitutes" for the mother or mothering functions. These seemingly insignificant objects may be imbued with symbolic meanings with which they are not inherently endowed. Tolpin (1972) elaborated on Winnicott's formulations, stating that a transitional object acts as a "soothing psychic structure." Deri (1978) said that the "transitional object establishes a bridge between the old and known and the new and unknown."

When a toddler forms an attachment to a teddy bear or a blanket, these objects come to represent the soothing functions of the mother. The use of objects for self-soothing during the normal separation-individuation process enables the child to tolerate ambivalence and to differentiate between the "me" and the "not me." When all else fails (i.e., mother is not available), the transitional objects tolerate the discharge of both negative and positive affects, thereby helping the child's developing sense of self. As the soothing functions of the object become internalized as part of the intrapsychic structure, the child becomes capable of self-soothing without the use of an object. The transitional object "enables the infant . . . to begin to achieve a degree of independence from the mother by virtue of his own mental activities—he has at hand a means to calm himself" (Tolpin 1972).

Coppolillo (1967) proposed that the use of transitional phenomena in the service of differentiation from the mother is a prerequisite to the development of a secure autonomous ego and makes up the greater part of the infant's experience. "Throughout life [these phenomena are] retained in the intense experiencing that belongs to the arts and to religion and to imaginative living and to creative scientific work" (Winnicott 1953).

In the course of development, the child relinquishes the original transitional object but not its qualities (Downey 1978). During adolescence, Downey (1978) adds, "there is a resurgence of, and re-emphasis on, the importance of transitional phenomena for psychological growth and development." Transitional phenomena are more apt to be "activities of the ego" aimed at mastering the revival of feelings of separateness from mother. Rather than use toys, adolescents may use their diaries as "actual and symbolic manifestations of particular mental operations having the aim of establishing a sense of mother at a 'not mother' time" (Downey 1978). The diary may also be used to unconsciously create a "not mother" realm in the service of differentiation. Adolescent transitional objects may be experienced as intensely as the toddler's blanket. Objects are endowed with "transitional qualities which will allow him or her a sense of safe conduct through adolescence'' (Downey 1978).

Transitional objects are used to promote development throughout the life cycle. At each successive stage, they reflect higher and more complex levels of differentiation and integration.

Clinical Data

Clinical material for this paper was drawn from a pilot study of seven women, aged eighteen to twenty-three, who had kept a diary between the ages of twelve and eighteen. Subjects were recruited through an advertisement; each participated in a three-hour interview. All came from middle-class families and represented a range of ethnic and religious backgrounds. They were asked to describe in detail their personal background, use of the diary, and feelings about the diary. The women submitted self-selected excerpts from their adolescent diaries. To avoid bias in their responses or their choice of excerpts, they were not informed of the specific focus of the study until after the interview was completed.

Results of the study support the claim that diary writing is a phase-appropriate developmental phenomenon. The findings suggest that the diary is an adjunct to, not a substitute for, real object relationships. It functions as a transitional object by generating calm, integrating affect and thought and facilitating differentiation. One subject said:

> It's so hard to separate yourself, and I think that's part of the diary's use. . . . When a girl starts writing a diary, she's discovering her own self and that discovery leads to the realization that, whether she knows it or not, she *is* separating herself from her family for the first time. The minute you start writing things down, you've separated yourself! Because you're suddenly keeping something—something tangible—from your parents.

At times of transition or crisis, the use of the diary may escalate in a way reminiscent of the toddler's heightened need for his or her transitional object:

> I wrote more frequently at times when I was having more confusion or anxiety, and when I was on trips.

It was being away from the physical home that made me write more. I'd write more frequently in times of extreme happiness or extreme crabbiness. I would often write directly after I'd had a fight with my mother. I would go to my room, burst into tears, and then begin to analyze it in my diary.

There may be such an intense connection to the object that the threat of losing the attachment creates significant anxiety. Fears that a parent might surreptitiously read the diary may be experienced not only as a threat of exposure of the diary's content but as an intrusion into the "intermediate area of experience" (Winnicott 1953).

Another excerpt reads:

I'm very protective about my journal. I really like my journal. I love the physical appearance of it—there's just so much of me in there. Even scribbling in it, it's just so cute! I always want to continue to have one. I love when I see the pages filling up. . . . I usually kept my diary hidden, but one day I went to school and I had left it out on the floor, and I had heart attacks all day because I knew that I had not hidden that diary. And I thought my mother will go in, and she'll see it and she'll read it. All day—I even went home from school early that day, I was so uptight about the whole idea.

Some of the subjects addressed their diaries as long-lost friends or lovers. At age fourteen, after a summer's hiatus from writing, one subject wrote:

Dear Understanding Ear, It's great to have you back even though it was I who booted you out. But I feel we can make a comeback. I won't call you "Understanding Ear" as much but you are once again in my heart and I love it.

Another wrote, at age fifteen:

Dearest! It has been too long! I have neglected you terribly. I can't help it. I'm kind of freaking out. I think about my childhood, my high school days, and next year. I'm going to do a lot of growing up. . . . I have the potential to become a fascinating adult—I just need a little experience.

One young woman developed an aesthetic attachment to her diary and was calmed by its mere presence:

I kept it on my desk and I had on top of it that Thoreau quote about how some men march to the beat of a different drummer done in calligraphy. It would sit in the middle of my desk, and when it was sitting there it meant that all was in good order. It was kind of important somehow.

The beginning process of internalization of the object and its qualities is illustrated in the following:

When I argued with my mother, I could tell myself things like, "Well, she's just going through menopause," or "she's trying to be sympathetic, but she doesn't understand my feelings." And then in the diary I would talk about how I felt about it. *It was kind of like being my own mother in a way.* [Emphasis added]

I called my diary "Meg" until I was 15. She definitely wasn't a part of me. . . . I thought I was writing to a real person! Then, around 15, I stopped addressing my entries to "Meg." I guess the diary became more like a part of *me,* who would help me figure things out.

The function of a diary as a self-soothing mechanism in adolescence is illustrated in the following:

It was calming . . . if I felt anxious or upset or angry, it was practically like taking a sedative. I would just sit down and force myself to write exactly what I felt. A lot of times I would feel angry, sad, or anxious and I really couldn't put my finger on what had me bothered. By sitting down and just outlining what was going on, it really almost always made me feel a lot better.

I was just able to talk to the diary . . . and it's been an incredible therapy ever since—when I'm upset I just write until I fall asleep. There's nothing better for depression than sleeping through it!

It was an immense relief to sit down and write. I don't know why

. . . it just made me feel better to sit down and have a friendly talk with myself even if it was about absolutely nothing. It got to be something I really looked forward to.

The diary as a transitional object in adolescence enters the sphere of object relations. The diary becomes a familiar, known extension of the emerging self and facilitates the negotiation of the adolescent passage. At age fifteen, a subject wrote in her diary:

I love these times of being alone with myself; I used to hate it and be lonely and afraid. But now I almost relish these special quiet times before human contact when I can think deeply, read, study, and just wallow in peacefulness.

A diary is an object the diarists sought when they felt besieged by confusing or intense emotions. Blos (1962) pointed to the diary's function as a place to release tensions that might otherwise lead to premature acting out. "Verbalization," he stated, "always brings mental content closer to the quality of realness. Living through experiences and emotions by putting them down in writing closes the door—at least partially and temporarily—to acting out." For the adolescent, the diary tolerates the discharge of *all* affects, while it employs the more highly developed ego functions characteristic of this phase of development. The subjects said:

It's a vent for the emotions. If you keep all these things bottled up inside you, well, it's kind of like when people say "I'll stop and count to ten before I blow up." In those ten seconds, you can pull yourself together and act like a rational person. So, instead of counting to ten, I'd write first, and then I could handle things on a much more intellectual level rather than just becoming emotionally nuts about the whole thing.

I had so many thoughts rattling around in my mind, I had to write some of them down or I was going to go completely bonkers. Even talking to my best friend, to whom I told everything, wasn't enough.

I probably would be dead if I hadn't written things down because when I saw myself getting into trouble, writing it down really made me realize, "Whoa! You've really got to stop!" It was like a safety valve. I think I would've turned violent, and I had a mouth like a sewer.

The relief the diarists experienced seems similar to that of a child who is reunited with her discarded blanket after angrily throwing it down a flight of stairs.

One diary entry, written by a sixteen-year-old, reflects the diary's sedating quality:

I've got to sit here and write for a while—my mind feels like it's falling apart and I feel I must take certain measures to reconstruct it. . . . What has happened to me and to all those who compose my world? I have grown conceited, complacent, and self-important, cynical, depressive, and possessive, yet I dislike myself intensely, lack confidence, feel continuously disturbed and long for faith, joy, and freedom. What am I becoming? Who am I? Why? [three pages later] I feel much better now, calmer, since I've written . . . it seems I have to be able to like myself before I can work toward self-expression and communication with others. . . .

At fourteen, a subject wrote of her confusion and ambivalence. Her entry is a poignant illustration of life between two worlds:

Dear Diary! It's been one hell of a time. I'm growing up you might say . . . and while I'm growing up, I have gotten the teenage tendency of wanting to be me—an individual, independent. Only I can't be, to a certain extent. Among my friends, my life is my own. Among my family, my life is theirs . . . together they meet and draw swords. It's a battle going on inside of me. Never ending. To tell you the truth, sometimes I think I'm going crazy.

Analysis of the diarists' retrospective reports and verbatim diary excerpts enhances our understanding of the diary-diarist relationship. The data strongly support the notion of the diary as a transitional object and point to its developmental function. These findings have implications for theory and practice.

Clinical Implications

Some fortunate young people pass through the phase of adolescence in a benign manner (Masterson 1975; Offer 1969); a great many do not. Difficulties in treating troubled adolescents are well documented in the literature (Blos 1962; Freud 1958; Meeks 1971; Schimel 1974). Often, the adolescent's psychic structure is in a state of turmoil. In psychotherapy, direct interpretation of unconscious and transferential material may threaten the patient's immature ego and contribute to resistance and acting-out behavior. It is important that the therapist allies with the adolescent's observing ego during the reorganization of defenses. Meeks (1971) advocated the therapeutic use of adolescent symbolic productions such as poetry, art, and stories as they may reveal valuable information regarding the adolescent's real concerns. He suggested that, if a patient brings a friend to a session, it may serve to lower the patients' anxiety and provide useful material for discussion.

The developmental issues outlined in this paper suggest that a diary can be a useful clinical tool, in keeping with Blos (1962), to aid in synthesis and mastery. Because of the unique nature of adolescent therapy, development of a positive transference may be problematic. Feelings and fantasies projected onto the diary may be explored to understand unconscious and transferential material that is otherwise unavailable. The adolescent who brings her diary to a therapy session may be, symbolically, bringing a "friend." Discussion of the diary-diarist relationship can shed light on the quality of her everyday interactions and concerns.

Summary

The concept of the diary as a transitional object adds a new perspective to the theory and treatment of adolescents. The findings of this pilot study suggest that the diary mirrors, soothes, helps inhibit frightening impulses, and helps integrate inner and outer realities. These functional aspects of the diary become internalized into the evolving psychic structure just as the analogous functions of the therapist in the context of a positive transference are internalized.

The use of the adolescent diary in psychotherapy enhances and enriches the meaning of the treatment alliance and promotes the progress of the "second separation-individuation." The therapist's sensitive and creative understanding of the diary-diarist relationship can lead to improved treatment strategies for adolescent patients. Further empirical research on the phenomenon of adolescent diary writing may deepen our clinical and theoretical understanding of this challenging population.

NOTE

I gratefully acknowledge Helene Cooper Jackson, Ph.D., L.I.C.S.W., for her valuable assistance in the preparation of this chapter.

REFERENCES

Baruch, G. K. 1968–1969. Anne Frank on adolescence. *Adolescence* 3:425–434.

Bernfeld, S. 1927 Present-day psychology of puberty. *Imago* 13:1–56.

Blos, P. 1962. *On Adolescence: A Psychoanalytic Interpretation.* New York: Free Press.

Blos, P. 1967. The second individuation process of adolescence. *Psychoanalytic Study of the Child* 22:162–186.

Coppolillo, H. P. 1967. Maturational aspects of the transitional phenomenon. *International Journal of Psycho-Analysis* 48:237–246.

Deri, S. 1978. Vicissitudes of symbolization and creativity. In S. Grolnick and L. Barkin, with W. Muensterberger, eds. *Between Reality and Fantasy.* New York: Jason Aronson.

Deutsch, H. 1944. *Psychology of Women.* Vol. 1. New York: Grune & Stratton.

Downey, T. W. 1978. Transitional phenomena in the analysis of early adolescent males. *Psychoanalytic Study of the Child* 33:19–46.

Elkind, D. 1971. Egocentrism in adolescence. In H. Thornburg, ed. *Contemporary Adolescence: Readings.* Belmont, Calif.: Brooks/Cole.

Frank, A. 1947. *The Diary of a Young Girl.* New York: Modern Library, 1952.

Freud, A. 1958. Adolescence. *Psychoanalytic Study of the Child* 13:255–278.

Gilligan, C. 1982. *In a Different Voice.* Cambridge, Mass.: Harvard University Press.

Group for the Advancement of Psychiatry. 1968. *Normal Adolescence: Its Dynamics and Impact.* Vol. 6, Report 68. New York: Scribner's.

Hug-Hellmuth, H. von. 1919. *A Young Girl's Diary.* New York: Barnes & Noble.

Kohlberg, L. 1981. *The Philosophy of Moral Development.* San Francisco: Harper & Row.

Kohut, H. 1971. *The Analysis of the Self.* New York: International Universities Press.

Masterson, J. 1975. The psychiatric significance of adolescent turmoil. In A. Esman, ed. *Psychology of Adolescence.* New York: International Universities Press.

Meeks, J. 1971. *The Fragile Alliance.* Baltimore: William & Wilkins.

Offer, D. 1969. Adolescent turmoil. In *The Psychological World of the Teenager—a Study of Normal Adolescent Boys.* New York: Basic.

Scarlett, G. 1971. Adolescent thinking and the diary of Anne Frank. *Psychoanalytic Review* 58:265–278.

Schimel, J. 1974. Two alliances in the treatment of adolescents: toward a working alliance with parents and a therapeutic alliance with the adolescent. *Journal of the American Academy of Psychoanalysis* 2:243–253.

Tolpin, M. 1972. On the beginnings of a cohesive self. *Psychoanalytic Study of the Child* 26:316–352.

Winnicott, D. W. 1953. Transitional objects and transitional phenomena. *International Journal of Psycho-Analysis* 34:89–97.

9   THE CONTRIBUTION OF PSYCHOANALYSIS TO THE PSYCHOTHERAPY OF ADOLESCENTS

PETER BLOS

Selected Principles of Adolescent Psychotherapy

Psychoanalysis is a theory of the human mind and a method of healing its ills. As a theory of the mind psychoanalysis has a bearing—either as a technique or as an explication—on all kinds of systematic endeavors to influence and change human behavior within the limit of the individual's wish to do so. True enough, this wish is not always present as our ready ally, and it becomes our job to induce a desire for change. What we can always rely on is the patient's wish to be relieved of an unpleasant mental state. But too often the deliverance from mental pain is expected to come about by that legendary recovery of a repressed childhood memory which has become the popular mystique of psychotherapy in many of its varieties. The romantic concept of therapy, so widespread today, is simply being "made to feel good." Contemporary language uses the word "therapy" with this kind of connotation in mind. People speak of going skiing, talking to a friend, or listening to music as "therapeutic," equating the experience of pleasure and relief from distress with the essence of the therapeutic process. Such expectations brush aside the fact that therapy not only resolves old conflicts but introduces by its very nature new conflicts which—by their continual resolution—lift psychic functioning onto a higher, more

A shorter version of this paper was presented at the first Institute of the Association for Child Psychoanalysis on "Child Therapy from an Analytic Perspective," San Diego, California, March 19, 1981.

complex level. This level, which we call maturity, can never be maintained easily and effortlessly. It is, assuredly, a life task.

The specific therapeutic endeavor of which I speak here is psychoanalytic psychotherapy of the adolescent. Its method, generally speaking, aims at restoring or advancing optimal psychic functioning in harmony with the self and the social world in which the patient lives. Contrary to the popular conception of psychotherapy, I think of optimal psychic functioning as encompassing the capacity to tolerate a modicum of anxiety and depression (Zetzel 1964), since both these disquieting affects are irreducible attributes of the human condition. Insight, in and by itself, does nothing; its therapeutic effectiveness always remains contingent on the use which the ego makes of it toward the expansion of its realm in mental life. The actuality of this expansion is reflected and observable within the contemplative and expressive interplay which flows ceaselessly between the self and the object world.

We are confronted initially in therapy with two basic variables: one refers to the manifestation of a psychological disturbance (be it a neurosis, a phobia, a delinquency, a social inadequacy, etc.); the other variable is reflected in the patient's thoughts or fantasies about therapy and the therapeutic situation. We have learned from psychoanalysis that resistance to change not only represents an impediment in the course of therapy but also denotes a healthy capacity of the psychic organism to protect an established and familiar way of functioning against outside interference. With the slow emergence of the therapeutic alliance the patient yields—ever so cautiously—to a restructuring of his personality organization. The conservation of the psychic status quo is reflected in specific self-preservative mental activities which we call "defenses." Both "resistance" and "defense" denote capabilities of the psychic apparatus which are basic and indispensable in human life; they protect the psychic organism against the infliction of injury or the incapacitation of functioning.

In order to ascertain the location of the elusive line of demarcation which divides normal from abnormal resistance and defense (in therapy and in life), psychoanalytic theory serves as a useful guide. To triangulate the line of demarcation, we must focus our attention simultaneously from three points of view. First, we investigate the patient's present condition; we refer to this as diagnosis or, less rigidly and more dynamically conceived, as assessment. Second, we explore the life history of the patient in order to discover enlightening clues for a more discriminating, that is, genetic, understanding of his present condition. Third, we compare both of these investigative efforts with an age-specific model or norm in order to determine the degree of deviation. In short, what I suggest here is a developmental approach to adolescent psychotherapy in order to improve the coordination of assessment and therapy. As is well known, in working with adolescents it is a most difficult task to tease out in the clinical picture what is a normal disturbance due to the developmental upheaval of the age and what constitutes a truly psychopathological condition. One of the inherent tasks of adolescent psychotherapy is to expose the adolescent to the painful recognition of inner conflict and of the illusions which a wished-for self tries to maintain. This transaction requires from the therapist the most genuine empathy, the most delicate tact, and the most firm and consistent attitude. In making this remark I hear the echo of an older adolescent's irate response to my reminding him that, even though he wished fervently to be a writer, the unalterable fact remained that he had never written more than a line—if that much. He shouted with a pleading desperation in his voice, "What is this? I thought you are supposed to make your patient feel good about himself." What motivated this adolescent to enter therapy was his desire to attain the narcissistic self-image of fame through the magic of therapy. The source of his failure in actively pursuing any goal lay camouflaged behind self-deceiving illusions. Confrontation with these irrationalities in his life represented the opening move in the emotional struggle called psychotherapy.

The note I struck in telling this incident leads me to a basic theme of adolescence. I have often been asked what, in my opinion, is the most difficult developmental task with which the adolescent has to cope. My answer has not always been the same, but years of experience have convinced me that the most painful task which faces the adolescent is the deidealization of self and object. With this statement I wish to convey the developmental fact that many of the narcissistic supplies which the young child receives from the "holding environment" (Winnicott 1965) are drying up with the advent of puberty. At this stage of the life cycle, biological and social demands are voiced relentlessly by the maturational process and urge the individual to renounce the infantile sources of emotional security. Similarly, the external sources of identity constancy and self-esteem regulation are to be replaced gradually by internal sources and by object relations of a different order. The new and extrafamilial object ties of the adolescent are not just replacements or displacements of infantile attachments; on the contrary, they are new creations, even though they contain elements of familiar object qualities. By the same token, they also reflect the exclusion or rejection of qualities which the familiar objects of childhood possessed. The adolescent does not simply replicate his past by repeating it either in fact or in disguise; rather, he actively employs his expanding mental and social resources to shape for himself a wider, more inclusive and exclusive surround by breaking through the bounds of the familiar patterns of his childhood. From a changed and changing body and surround the adolescent receives and elicits an array of novel and untested sensations and stimulations via a widening and more complex interaction system between the self and the object world. This process, if vigorously sustained by the individual and his surround, furnishes those developmental activators necessary for keeping in motion the adolescent's forward thrust toward adulthood. I must leave the itinerary of this developmental journey unexplored on this occasion because issues more urgent to the topic of this chapter require attention.

We know from the work of Mahler, Pine, and Bergman (1975) that the young child passes through a phase of psychic structure formation designated as "individuation." Briefly, this process encompasses the period when the toddler—from early to late toddlerhood—internalizes the caretaking person or persons, usually the mother, and thus acquires object representations which possess an internally available object presence. Obviously, this acquisition of psychic structure memorializes the virtues as well as the flaws of the object world as it was originally experienced. We must not ignore the fact that these early internalizations remain under ceaseless scrutiny by the ego, whose work is governed progressively by the growing influence of the reality principle. To the extent that this process is successful, the autonomy of the ego gains in scope and, by the same token, the ego's dependency on the environment diminishes. Concomitantly, the line of demarcation between fantasy and reality becomes drawn not only more sharply but also more indelibly.

Mental and sexual maturation requires an overhauling of internalizations, identifications, and object relations. These changes are effected or practiced via social ritualizations; among these we refer to social role assignments as powerful agents in the adolescent's life. I have formulated these internal changes, designated as the "structural reorganization of the adolescent personality," in dynamic terms as the "second individuation process of adolescence" (Blos 1967). The first individuation facilitated the young child's existence as a demarcated psychological entity through the internalization of the caretaking persons and the impinging surround. Thus, psychic structure formation takes its origin. We can discern the consolidation of nuclei of the self around which experience becomes organized. These are the steps in psychic differentiation which afford the young child a forward move toward physical independence; the internalized objects have become the guardians of the self or the protectors against abandonment anxiety.

In contrast to the infantile individuation process just outlined, the second individuation process represents the adolescent task of achieving independence from the internalized objects and their early formative influence on ego and superego. These internal changes not only effect the normative adolescent personality transformations but also account for much of the proverbial emotional turbulence of this age. The second individuation process proceeds either noisily and agitatedly or calmly and silently vis-à-vis the surrounding world and the self-observing ego. In any case, we witness often enough affective states and forms of behavior which are abnormal or bizarre. Adolescent abnormalities, emotional and behavioral, can best be assessed as to their transient or irreversible nature by viewing the disturbance in the light of adolescent psychic restructuring. The unavailability of the accustomed and dependable internal stabilizers of childhood seems to be responsible for many of the typical and transient personality characteristics of this age. Since every therapist is well acquainted with them, I refer to them only briefly by mentioning the swing from avid object hunger to bleak object avoidance and emotional withdrawal; from motoric impulsivity and action craving to lassitude and limp indifference; from the idealization of ideas or heroes to cold egotistical cynicism; from narcissistic self-sufficiency, imperviousness, and arrogance to the depressive and dejected state of shame and guilt. We always find one or the other of these characteristics in the clinical picture of adolescent psychopathology, regardless of whether it is definitive, namely, irreversible by development, or it accompanies development and is therefore transient in nature and self-liquidating in time. The unrelenting malfunction of the adolescent personality is the sign of a miscarriage of the adolescent process, namely, the failure to yield adaptively to the challenges of the second individuation process.

Paradoxically, progressive development during adolescence requires the capacity to regress in order to rework those infantile tasks which had been too taxing to master at the tender age of early childhood. At the advanced age of adolescence the tasks have to be dealt with anew by an ego that has acquired in the intervening years a resourcefulness commensurate to the task of the second individuation process. Internal conflicts, manifest in adolescent mental disturbances, lie within a defensive spectrum which extends from the irresistible urgency to regress to the frantic forward thrust into adultomorphic behavior, thus sidestepping a developmental progression that requires *time* to lend firmness and durability to psychic restructuring. Transient regressive movements are characteristic for this task and are at no period of life as obligatory as during the adolescent process. I have designated this regresssion "regression in the service of development" (Blos 1967). Clinical observation renders the differentiation between normal regression and pathological regression at adolescence a knotty and puzzling problem. I have found that a discriminating review of the individual life history will throw light on the diagnostic and prognostic understanding of the case at hand. Let us admit that we are often reluctant to say that an adolescent does not require therapeutic attention when his or her behavior is a cause of concern to parents, teachers, and the community; we are equally hesitant and cautious not to err in the opposite direction. At such critical junctures we turn for clarification to the dynamic conceptualizations of development which psychoanalytic psychology offers us.

At this point I shall shift the focus of my presentation from a theoretical to a clinical one. The case I shall present not only exemplifies my antecedent remarks but also opens up new territory in which to advance the exploration of our topic. I have chosen this case because it demonstrates the clinical usefulness of psychoanalytic theory in the field of psychotherapeutic work regardless of its official designation, which might be psychotherapy, casework, or child guidance. In the context of this discussion I pay attention to the application of psychoanalytic principles to the treatment of the adolescent outside the treatment modality of psychoanalysis proper.

I have selected a case of psychoanalytic psychotherapy because the vast majority of disturbed adolescents are treated—if treated at all—by this treatment modality. I also wish to demonstrate my conviction that a psychoanalytically grounded comprehension of a case influences more decisively and favorably the conduct and outcome of therapy than does the frequency of weekly sessions. The intensity of therapy is by no means proportionate to the frequency of therapeutic contacts. Which treatment modality is finally chosen as the treatment of choice is ideally determined by the assessment of the presenting disturbance, but in clinical practice extraneous factors affect the decision, such as the ability to pay, the patient's psychological accessibility, or the therapist's geographical accessibility. This consideration does not deny the indisputable fact that a certain kind of emotional illness requires a specific treatment modality in order to effect cure. Even though we wish to render a perfect match between type of illness and treatment modality, we must admit that reality factors often taint the purity of our principled judgment. Every clinician has discovered to his surprise that a judicious recourse to what, pejoratively, is called a "compromise" of treatment choice might bring about a remarkable amelioration of the presenting disturbance. It has been my experience that this kind of rewarding outcome can occur most often when treatment is undertaken during the stages of primary development, namely, during the years of preadult life (Blos 1970).

The Case of Mary

The patient on whom I shall report was seen over a period of five months in individual sessions once a week.

Mary, a fifteen-year-old girl, was brought to my attention by her parents. She was an only child. From the description the parents gave me of their daughter's troubles emerged the typical clinical picture of an agoraphobia in an adolescent girl. This condition had for some time exerted a seriously confining influence on her life. She was unable to leave her home and walk on the street without being accompanied by her mother or a girl friend. The companion had to be female. She felt uncomfortable or actually anxious in the presence of males if they were older than herself. Being in the company of her father made her apprehensive and uneasy. She had confided to her mother the fear of men which possessed her and over which she had no control.

Mary attended a parochial girls' school with only women teachers. Once inside the school building she felt safe, was anxiety free, and enjoyed the time with her many friends. However, after school Mary's life was restricted to her home. She never visited a friend unless picked up by a companion; she never visited her beloved grandfather in the country where she had spent many happy times when she was younger. In fact, for several years she had shunned his company. The parents had observed over the last year a drop in her academic work and also a

110

detached, morose, and worried moodiness. Mary was particularly nasty and impertinent to her mother on whom she depended not only for traveling to and from school but for all her movements outside her home. She accused her parents of hating her, of wanting to get rid of her, and of wishing her out of the house. While she hurled such accusations at her parents, she never believed a word of them to be true. The mother was a hardworking, caring, and proper woman who was closely attached to her daughter; the father was a responsible provider, even though he displayed at times a flighty, impulsive, and self-indulging disposition. During the prephobic period Mary looked neither right nor left when walking alone to school but kept staring at a static object like a building, a billboard, or the pavement, always sensing around herself the presence of men, whether or not they actually were there. It is reasonable to assume that in these situations men were constantly on her mind without being associated with any conscious mental content. In fact, Mary was a reserved and shy girl who behaved in public with extraordinary decorum.

I shall now report a secret which Mary had told her mother one and a half years earlier with the explicit request never to tell her father. This secret—so I later discovered—was to be of crucial importance for the understanding of the case. The secret which the mother reported to me in the initial—and only—interview I had with the parents was a memory that had troubled the girl for a long time, but more persistently during the last several years. When she was about four years old, so Mary remembered, she was in her parents' bed as was the family custom on Sunday mornings. That particular morning the mother was already up, dressed, and ready to go out. Mary and her father were fooling around in bed, when she suddenly heard her mother say in a stern voice, "You do that only with your wife." This phrase struck like a bolt of lightning and stayed silently in her mind until she repeated it to her mother some ten years later.

Mary entered psychotherapy with the determination to get well. Should her mother be unable to bring her to my office, she would arrange to travel with one of her girl friends. Mary unburdened herself eagerly of her thoughts, experiences, and memories which had lain buried in her mind since early childhood. She told me that for the last two years she had avoided being in the presence of her father. "Even though I love him," she said, "I don't like to be in his company or near him; often I hate him." She talked freely about her romantic, childish daydreams or about the troubled times of her childhood. Lately she often cried when alone in her room listening to sentimental music, or she sat brooding over her parents' unhappy marriage. She described quite graphically her father's drunken binges, his coming home late at night with the help of an unfamiliar woman, shouting, cursing, and toppling over furniture. She remembered well the sights, the sounds, and her hate of the other woman who—so she thought—had degraded her father.

In the course of talking about herself Mary told me "the secret" which she had confided to her mother. She began her narrative by saying that on Sunday mornings "I used to cuddle with my parents in their bed. That day I asked my dad to put his arm around me, when I heard my mother say—she was just ready to leave the room and go out—'You do that only with your husband!' " After a pause Mary continued, "Not until I was ten years old did the meaning of that remark become clear to me; I knew then it had something to do with sex, love, and necking."

As soon as Mary had finished telling me her secret, I realized that her version was different from the one reported to me by her mother. Let me point out the discrepancy between the two stories. In one, as told to me by Mary's mother, the girl had heard her childhood mother say, "You do that only with your wife." In the version Mary told me she had heard her childhood mother say, "You do that only with your husband." In the first comment the father stands accused; in the second, Mary is the guilty one. In both statements the child heard herself addressed in the forbidden role of a presumptive marriage partner. Both role arrogations represented for Mary a psychic reality of traumatic consequences. What the girl had heard was the mother's accusation that the father loves his little girl as he loves his wife, or, in other words, that he desires forbidden sexual relations with his little daughter. The enigmatic sentence, etched indelibly in her memory, had acquired elaborate and formidable meanings with the advancing years of puberty.

The self-accusatory and guilty state, implicit in Mary's version, was confirmed by her through a dream in which she kisses a man who is a distant relative. Mary explained, "I hardly know him and I really do not like him," adding quickly that she was related to him "by marriage only and not by blood." To my astonishment she was acutely surprised by the fact that in the dream it was she (not the man) who made the sexual advance by kissing him. Via this nonincestuous and nonattractive man in the dream she came to acknowledge the sexual wishes and fantasies which—so we had good reason to assume—lay hidden behind the phobic symptom.

Her reaction to the dawning awareness of her sexual memories, fantasies, and wishes which she had shared with me was a surprising one. For the next session Mary arrived "dressed to kill." From under a shock of blond hair, fluffed up into a spectacular aura, there peeked out a child's face, painted clumsily with rouge, lipstick, and mascara. Tight, white sailor pants completed her shapely appearance, which amounted to a caricature of a juvenile make-believe streetwalker. I shall return to the patient's sexual acting out in the transference when I arrive at the discussion of the case.

Let me state at this point that the discrepancy between the two versions of the "secret"—we will never know for certain which is the true one[1]—made me form the hunch that the different versions represented the opposing sides of the mental conflict which had become manifest in the phobia. I therefore decided to bring the version told to me by the mother to Mary's attention,[2] thus making her aware of the fact that two versions of the secret existed simultaneously, but in a dissociated state, in her mind. I expected from this intervention that her realization of the bewildering disparity would activate the synthesizing faculty of the ego. This psychic effort, so I reasoned, might bring about an active striving toward the resolution of a conflict which had been kept in mental limbo by the irreconcilable content of a memory whose double-faced nature was the cause of a pathological accommodation, namely, symptom formation. As was to be expected, Mary felt gradually less anxious and socially less constrained.

At this point the summer vacation intervened. I saw Mary again after an interval of two months. She had stayed at home during the beginning of her vacation until she realized that her mother had "too much of a need for my company." It was then that she decided to accept an invitation to her grandfather's house in the country where she had not visited for two years. She stayed with him for three weeks. With joy and pleasure she summed up her stay by saying, "I had a real good time." She experienced no anxiety when outdoors alone. She made friends, boys and girls, and became romantically attached to a boy from the village neighborhood. Since she returned home and started school, Mary was free of her phobic symptom. She was no longer in need of a companion on the street. On some days she preferred her girl friend to pick her up rather than meet her at an appointed place. On weekends she played golf with her father.

Mary seemingly had lost her symptom as smoothly and completely as a snake slithers out of its skin. Emotional transformations do not occur in this fashion. Simultaneous with the symptomatic improvement, Mary's demands on her mother became more exacting and frenzied, leading to passionate love-and-hate arguments. The mother reacted with resentment and hurt to Mary's bullying and demandingness; to this the girl responded with wild accusations of the mother's unkindness and lack of love. She burst into teary complaints about the cold indifference she received from her mother for the many pleasures Mary provided for her, such as cleaning the house in order to cheer her up on her return from work. Obviously, Mary's accounts of her dutiful household chores were wild distortions and exaggerations within the typical emotional struggle between an adolescent girl and her mother. In resentful anger Mary told me that she would no longer ask her mother to accompany her to school, "even if it kills me."

With the decline of the phobic symptom I saw the discord between mother and daughter mount and move into the center of Mary's emotional life. She was now engaged in a conflict with her mother, finding herself unable to face the intensity of her ambivalence at this stage of her postphobic psychic restructuring. I was therefore not surprised when she told me of her wish to terminate treatment. I decided to put no obstacle in the way of her decision, even though the mother was pleading for a continuation of therapy. A talk with the mother had convinced me that Mary's growing independence had aroused in her an anxious feeling of loneliness and estrangement. In the wish that Mary continue therapy I suspected her intention to use Mary's therapy as a way to preserve unaltered the close bond of emotional attachment between mother and child. This dimension added weight to my decision to let her terminate treatment at this juncture.

Discussion

The discussion of this case has the express purpose of extracting from it certain psychoanalytic principles which have an applicability far beyond the treatment of Mary. My first comment dwells on the human faculty of listening. It is common knowledge that the psychoanalyst's most time-consuming interaction with the patient is listening. In using the word "interaction" I attribute to the therapist's listening an active, not merely a receptive, quality. This kind of listening provides the therapist with information which is conveyed unintentionally by the patient and lies beyond what is literally communicated. The trained faculty of hearing what is communicated by the patient without his conscious awareness lifts the act of listening onto a special plane quite remote from the receptivity of a naturally good listener. Under the tutelage of a psychoanalytic orientation, listening is done by an educated ear. Theodore Reik (1948) has felicitously called it "listening with the third ear." This kind of listening proceeds in a state of suspended judgment which we call "free-floating attention." Content and sequence of the patient's communications are constantly viewed against the backdrop of psychoanalytic theory, or, in other words, they are perceived in association with multiple references, be they of a dynamic, genetic, adaptive, or developmental nature. While listening, the clinician elaborates hypothetical formulations in his mind, letting the clinical evidence that follows render the verdict whether or not the tentative construct was accurate. The therapist should be pleased with whatever the verdict might be, because it brings the truth closer to his reach. In addition, the therapist listens simultaneously to his own inner promptings which never fail to be elicited by the help-seeking individual as a patient and as a person. These promptings receive their buoyancy from the therapist's personal associative sensitivities, thus evoking in him a state of empathy. The voice of empathy is listened to with the same discriminating ear as is the voice of the patient, thus making audible—by a kind of mutual enforcement—what is often too faint a sound to be perceived in the patient's direct communications. From the multitude of these perceptions in the field of listening and observing there emerges insight into the patient's psychological state; based on this information we formulate guidelines for our therapeutic work. The point just outlined is illustrated in Mary's case by the elucidation of the secret as the vortex of a conflictual turbulence which was brought under control pathologically by her symptom. The insight into the content and dynamics of the secret pressed on me various therapeutic lines from which to choose.

During the entire course of therapy we constantly grope for reliable guidelines, particularly at certain way stations which challenge our clinical sagacity. At such times we project before our mental eye the whole therapeutic encounter in order to determine the direction into which treatment should move. This process scrutinizes not only how therapy has progressed so far but also what to expect from its continuation and where its limitations might lie. For an illustration of this point I refer to my assent to Mary's decision to terminate treatment.

Why did I do this? I did it after I had carefully juxtaposed the relative reasons for and against continuation of therapy. What weighed heavily in this act of decision making were the considerations which prompted me initially to take this girl in psychotherapy. After a brief acquaintance I could see that Mary was a deeply troubled girl, anxious rather than depressed or emotionally withdrawn. Her reaching out for help was genuine, and her therapeutic cooperation could be engaged. Furthermore, I formed the opinion that her phobia was a symptom in formation, partially still operating on the level of acting out a fantasy. In other words, the conflict was not yet fully internalized; it had not yet progressed to the state of a neurotic condition but was still on the way toward consolidation into a structured symptom. Her emotional illness was still enmeshed in the adolescent process and accessible to psychotherapy. It seemed to me that the testing of this preliminary assessment was an effort worth undertaking.

It is noteworthy that in the treatment of Mary a phase of "working through" was not discernible, even though this phase supposedly brings treatment to its successful and natural conclusion. Two comments are in order at this point. Whenever treatment is undertaken while development is still in potential progress, it remains the aim of psychotherapy to bring impeded development into flux and redirect it into the mainstream of adaptive growth. Furthermore, I wish to emphasize the incongruous fact that during adolescence therapeutic achievement becomes manifest not only by a symptomatic improvement and a more satisfactory performance in life generally but also by the appearance of a new wave of disturbances; these, however, are now of a developmentally more phase-adequate nature. In Mary's case, this turn was signaled by her forward thrust into an active social and academic participatory life and by the appearance of an acute daughter-mother conflict. These adaptations are usually compromise formations which will serve the adolescent well enough to move toward a reasonably satisfactory closure of adolescence. In cases where this goal remains out of reach, we must conclude that another therapeutic modality is indicated.

Pursuing the lines of thought I have just sketched, I wish to make a further remark about Mary's recovery. When the phobic symptom was abating, I observed that the focus of her disturbance had shifted to a regressive acting out of a typical mother-daughter ambivalence struggle. This reengagement in preoedipal dependency and attachment issues represents a normal and transient stage in female adolescence. In

Mary's case it was kept in abeyance by the fixation on the oedipal level. However, we must not overlook that the passionate turn to the oedipal father provided simultaneously a bulwark against the regressive pull to the mother of early childhood, the preoedipal mother. This typical, that is, normative, regressive pull in female adolescence usually gives rise to all kinds of attachment and dependency needs as well as to rebellious and distancing behavior. Seeing the developmental picture in this light, one might have been inclined to offer Mary's liberated emotions an opportunity to find their adolescent-adequate balance with the help of continued psychotherapy. However, as my therapeutic stance indicates, I elected in this adolescent case to suspend treatment after a reasonable resumption of a developmental flux or reengagement had been attained. This I did with the thought in mind that treatment might be resumed if another insurmountable impasse were to arise in the course of her growing up. We could well speak here of an age-appropriate therapy delivered in installments. The risk of leaving the therapeutic work incomplete has to be gauged against the benefits of an autonomous developmental advance; this in turn furnishes that confidence and trust in therapeutic work which are necessary for its resumption whenever a decisive need for it should arise.

Some readers may have wondered why I had neglected—if neglect it was—to deal with the girl's acting out in the therapy situation or—to be more precise—in the transference. I refer here to the session in which Mary appeared "dressed to kill." Her exhibitionistic and seductive behavior was obviously for my benefit. In order to explain my nonintervention I must mention the fact that my work with adolescent girls has taught me the paradoxical lesson that the interpretation of sexual acting out in the transference, done with the purpose of rendering sexual fantasies or wishes conscious and consequently subject to ego control and insight, quite to the contrary stimulates sexual excitation, which in turn provokes other forms of acting out such as, for instance, absenteeism or breaking off treatment. A complication of this nature becomes particularly virulent if the therapist is a man.

Acting out in the transference, as demonstrated by Mary's behavior when she appeared for her session "dressed to kill," presents a most delicate situation which has to be approached with utmost tact, sensitivity, and circumspection. A forthright interpretation should be given only if a breakdown of therapy is imminent due to a persevering and unmodulated, that is, direct, sexual transference. This cautiousness is suggested by the fact that the adolescent girl who develops a rapid and massive sexual transference to a male therapist equates his talking about transferential sexual feelings, wishes, and fantasies with his seductive intentions—indeed, with his desire for sexual intimacy with his female patient. The projective component of this reaction is obvious. While we are familiar with the ease and casualness with which most contemporary adolescents discuss matters of sex, it is noteworthy that the taboo—encompassing guilt, embarrassment, and shame—of incestuous emotions, when they come to life in the transference, has not lost any of its original stringency. Indeed, the adolescent state of sexual freedom has not at all affected this infantile realm.

Returning once more to Mary's transference behavior, I wish to emphasize that, in avoiding an interpretation of her acting out in the transference, I gave expression to my opinion that the resolution of her symptom would be feasible by pursuing her pathogenetic past without exposing to the light of awareness the sexual arousal in the transference. I attempted therefore to affect Mary's sexual acting out in the transference by helping her to rework, namely, resolve, the emotional conflict she had once experienced in the parental bed. My knowledge of the secret had laid out the path into this festering region of her mind. At any rate, by this incongruous therapeutic twist the usual direction of analytic technique was reversed. I succeeded in bringing the repressed component of her infantile conflict to her attention by using a lost memory that was recovered by outside information. I was persuaded to take this course because the concrete treatment situation had re-established the original triadic constellation with both Mary and therapist alone in the consulting room and the mother in the nearby waiting room as an absentee participant. This treatment approach was further strengthened by the fact that Mary possessed an unusually clear memory of her childhood and was in vivid touch with her pathogenetic past. It should be noted here that the particular kind of acting out in the transference which I described was never repeated.

In this connection I want to comment on the puzzling fact that Mary entered treatment—and indeed a productive one—with a man. Her phobia presented no hindrance to her therapeutic engagement; quite the contrary, it rather seemed to help it along. As hinted at above, on a psychological level, Mary was never alone with me during her visits to my office; the presence of her mother in the waiting room completed the triadic constellation in which her pathology was embedded. The *dramatis personae* were all in their proper places: they replicated the traumatic experience and set the stage for the fateful drama of early life to unfold in therapy. What might have eased this psychological trans-figuration with a male therapist was perhaps his advanced age; it blended, so to speak, oedipal passions with a more benign grandfather transference.[3]

There remains one more observation to be made. The symptom was never dealt with directly as a focal entity. The obvious and painful pathological condition, the phobia, was treated with a kind of atten-tional neglect. This therapeutic attitude is based on psychoanalytic theory and practice which have taught us that a neurotic symptom exists only as long as an unresolved conflict requires its presence; the function of the symptom can be seen in protecting the sense of self and in preventing catastrophic anxiety from flooding the psychic organism. By laying open the discrepancy in the two versions of Mary's secret, I exposed her divided self in front of her mental eye. By confrontation rather than by offering an interpretation of the phobic symptom—the dynamics of which were well understood—I made the dissociated drive components (embodied in the two versions of "I want you" vs. "you want me") available to the synthetic work of the ego. I expected from this effort that the patient would structure a conflictual organization of a different order than the pathological one—the phobia—which was built on repression, displacement, and projection. The endeavor just outlined was followed by an abatement of the phobia. Concomitantly, the conflictual focus shifted into the realm of the dyadic, preoedipal phase. With this shift Mary had attained a second chance to complete some of the unfinished business of her early childhood. Should she be equal to this adolescent task, I expected that she would be able to move into adult life less impeded and burdened by her past.

Follow-Up

The case of Mary would be left incomplete if there were no follow-up attached to it. Too many questions were raised, too many prognostic and alternative hunches were advanced for silence to descend at this point on Mary's posttherapeutic development. Our curiosity is justifi-ably directed to the specific ways in which therapy had affected her life.

Before Mary left my office at the end of our last session, we agreed that she would get in touch with me in the near future "just to let me know how she was getting along." For a long time I did not hear from her. Half a year had passed when I got a call from her saying that she wanted to see me. When we met it was as if no time had elapsed. She was obviously happy to see me again. She admitted readily that she had avoided me because she was afraid that being in my office or in my presence would bring to life all the memories she had shared with me and wanted to forget. She told me that she had not been able to manage her life as well as she had expected and would like to resume therapy.

In the following report I shall summarize Mary's life since I had seen her last and as told by her in the initial interview after her return. I shall focus on the use of this information in assessing whether a second installment of treatment was indicated.

Mary reported that she had experienced pleasant changes on three fronts of her life: (1) she and her mother had come closer together ("We can talk about everything and we enjoy each other's company. My mother has become my best friend"), (2) she had been out on several dates, and (3) she had improved remarkably in school. The gentle climate of family closeness recently was blown away by a tornado of family fights which always culminated in Mary's accusation to her mother, "You don't love me!" The emotional intensity of these fights inspired Mary's decision to see me. Although I was not able to elicit the cause or provocation of these fights, it was clear that the fighting made Mary dejected and miserable to the point that she felt compelled to make peace with her mother at any price. Mary reported that she was now on reasonably good terms with her father but felt "uncomfortable and uneasy" when greeted by him "with hugs and kisses" on his return from work.

Mary expressed great dislike of her tendency to daydream and had made efforts to counteract it by doing something or being in her mother's company. She used her room less as a refuge from the world or as a place to cry, sulk, and pity herself. However, she reported spells of moodiness; she said, "They just come and go without any rhyme or reason. But I feel much happier now than before I came to see you." She voiced the wish to be more like the girls of her age and "have fun" while decidedly disapproving of their preoccupation—in thought and deed—with sex. "My generation moves too fast" she said, and "I'm really afraid of guys." Within her rather proper social conduct the fact that two weeks prior to her revisiting me she had gotten drunk at her girl friend's birthday party stood out like an unaccountable apparition from the unknown.

While the street phobia was no longer a source of trouble, Mary still moved outdoors with a certain restraint; for example, she would not pass the corner filling station on her street because the men there could be counted on to whistle at her. She added, "I am quite prudish." However, she now could walk by herself to and from school as well as go downtown to do her shopping.

At this point we have to ask ourselves how the life-history data, covering the last six months, can be translated into an assessment of Mary's present psychological status and be used for the purpose of defining changes in her functioning which would speak clearly for or against the resumption of treatment. What struck me in Mary's account was the keen alertness of her self-observing ego. In contrast to her previous grasp of causality, namely, her pathological use of projection, she was now able to realize that the origin of her various emotional discomforts was internal. Furthermore, her wish to return to therapy signified that her first acquaintance with treatment had been a positive experience; in others words, she had invested the therapeutic process with a sense of trust and confidence. She could now separate her relatedness to the therapist and his function to help her from the therapist as a sexual being, a man. In other words, her response and attitude to the father figure (imago) and its reexperience in the outer world had become more discriminating and complex.

In an effort to strengthen her ego autonomy she had abstained actively from the self-indulgence in daydreams and self-pity. Her florid fantasy life had become ego alien. She had become determined "to do things," one of which was academic work, with the result that she had received praise and was considered a success by teachers and parents alike. Thus, she had created for herself a source of legitimate narcissistic pleasure. She literally beamed as an answer when I asked her, "Do you enjoy the A's on your report card?" In an effort to gain ego control over situations which she had previously avoided owing to anxiety arousal, she had faced them head-on: she had accepted dates and gone out. These friendships were short-lived in most instances because she became frightened by the erotic physical contact which the boys demanded. As a result she stayed away from them. This defeat on her first foray into heterosexual sociability had thrown Mary back into closeness to her mother. She was now caught between the desire to return to the safety of her home and the desire to enter the enviable world in which her peers moved. At one point in the interview I asked her what, in her opinion, was her present trouble? She answered without hesitation, "My insecurity." At the first stage of treatment the answer would have been a description of her phobia.

Mary's answer, "My insecurity," I shall now define in dynamic terms. It is evident from the clinical picture that the girl's ego proved incompetent to deal with the emotional tasks of adolescence. The gratification of any sexual urge from holding hands to kissing (such was the extent of her love life) had to be renounced entirely (so to say, *en bloc*) owing to the unreliability of her ego as a protector of her moral and physical integrity. This conflict was subjectively experienced by Mary as "insecurity." Her mental state was of the neurotic modality. In essence, Mary's illness was due to the tension between opposing wishes or needs, irreconcilable in their nature. I call attention to the juxtaposition of her getting drunk and being her mother's good little girl. This impasse or bind had by now congealed into an emotional and behavioral pattern which can best be described as an oscillating state between regressive and progressive trends and movements. This was the condition in which Mary reentered therapy. Because of the first stage of treatment, an advance in the internalization of conflict was noted; this change rendered Mary a promising candidate for the resumption of psychotherapy. However, the tale of that enterprise must wait to be told at another occasion.

Before I leave the follow-up of Mary I wish to make some general comments on this subject. I consider a follow-up of particular significance and urgency in all treatment reports concerning children or adolescents. This opinion is based on the fact that child and adolescent therapy, when undertaken while childhood development is still in progress, operates within given delimitations. These delimitations are conceived of as integral aspects of child development itself and lie beyond the particular effectiveness of a given therapeutic enterprise and its unique partnership. Therapy during childhood and adolescence can neutralize[4] the noxiousness of pathogenetic nuclei, formed early in life, only up to the developmental level or, more exactly, up to its potential normative presence (i.e., age) which the patient has attained at the time of treatment. Under the most fortunate circumstances the child emerges from therapy with a restored ego competence which proves equal to the developmental challenges that lie ahead. But we can never be certain whether new developmental tasks will not be found too taxing, in which case symptom formation—not necessarily symptom repetition—may be resumed.[5] In other words, we can never be certain whether a new developmental thrust will not activate pathogenetic remnants or residues that have survived the earlier therapeutic work.[6] The so-called and misnamed failures of child therapy are rarely predictable, especially after a satisfactory completion of therapy during preadult life.

It is an empirical fact that a large number of children who were treated successfully during childhood or adolescence resume therapy later in their lives. Follow-up studies promise to be of invaluable help for comprehending more clearly the delimitations inherent in child psychotherapy and child psychoanalysis. Even if follow-up studies cannot be pursued systematically, I suggest that they be undertaken randomly (as in the case of Mary), because they add a worthwhile edge of discriminating foresight and humility to any clinician's skill.

This brings my discussion to an end. The nature of the case chosen for illustration determined the selective attention to certain clinical issues drawn from the vast borderland that lies between psycho-analysis and psychoanalytically oriented psychotherapy. I am certain that many a reader wished I had given more attention to one or the other theoretical or technical problem. But, even though I could not fully attend to the topical richness of the subject under discussion, I nevertheless hope I conveyed and strengthened the conviction that the judicious use of psychoanalytic knowledge enhances significantly the scope and effectiveness of our psychotherapeutic work with adoles-cents.

NOTES

1. I was prepared to discover that both versions were auditory pro-jections of guilt with a delusional realness that remained attached to the memory.

2. The reader must have noticed that I committed an indiscretion when I quoted to Mary from my interview with her parents. It must have been obvious to her that her mother had reported the secret to me in front of her father, thus having broken the promise of silence the mother had given her daughter who requested it. In spite of all these considerations, I did not hesitate to use the therapeutic potential of the double-faced secret and run the risk of complicating and perhaps aborting the good work with the patient by involving the parents at this point in her treatment. I was confident that the therapeutic alliance was strong enough to ride out safely any emotional storm in case Mary should take me or her mother to task. As it turned out, none of these

complications came to pass. The girl was too profoundly occupied with past traumatic events to bother with their faint reverberations in the present.

3. Mary's first move away from her parental home was a prolonged vacation visit at her beloved grandfather's house which she had avoided for several years. It should be mentioned that the grandfather was a single man, a widower.

4. Within the framework of the structural theory we refer to this process in terms of stages in conflict resolution.

5. In such an instance the normative developmental task is comparable to a trauma inflicted on the psychic organism. In these instances, the trauma coalesces with dormant pathogenetic residues.

6. I am fully aware of the fact that development is not restricted to the period of childhood but is an ongoing process during the life cycle. But I submit that, within this broad spectrum, the developmental stages of preadult life are of an order that differs distinctly, in terms of the internalization of prototypical experiences and their effect on psychic structure formation, from that of the stages following later in life.

REFERENCES

Blos, P. 1967. The second individuation process of adolescence. *Psychoanalytic Study of the Child* 22:162–186.

Blos, P. 1970. *The Young Adolescent*. New York: Free Press.

Mahler, M. S.; Pine, F.; and Bergman, A. 1975. *The Psychological Birth of the Human Infant*. New York: Basic.

Reik, T. 1948. *Listening with the Third Ear*. New York: Farrar, Straus.

Winnicott, D. W. 1965. *Maturational Processes and the Facilitating Environment*. New York: International Universities Press.

Zetzel, E. R. 1964. Symptom formation and character formation. *International Journal of Psycho-Analysis* 45:151–157.

10 THE ADOLESCENT SELF DURING THE PROCESS OF TERMINATION OF TREATMENT: TERMINATION, INTERRUPTION, OR INTERMISSION?

RUDOLF EKSTEIN

Freud (1913) once suggested that the beginning and end phases of psychoanalysis can be taught as easily as the beginning and end phases of the royal game of chess. It is, he said, the middle game of chess, or the middle game of psychoanalysis, which can be learned only by observing a master. Freud's comment refers to the teaching and learning problems of the analytical process: the beginning of the analysis, the establishment of the therapeutic alliance and the therapeutic situation, the development of the transference neurosis, and, finally, the working through of the end phase. However, I suggest that in the treatment of adolescents it is the end phase which creates specific difficulties. It is seldom that psychotherapists describe their treatment of adolescent cases in terms of the kind of end treatment which gives the feeling of completion, of having reached the goal of treatment—the cure, the end point of the process.

In a previous article (1965), rather than put the emphasis on the point of termination, I described the termination *process*. I stressed the working through of the end phase as an important task in addition to the one of establishing criteria for ending.

Analytical work with adolescents (and this is also true for children) differs in one special respect from work with adults. Adults come to us with problems and symptoms of disturbed functioning. The task of the

Presented at the Hampstead Child Therapy Course and Clinic, London, June 30, 1982.

125

analytical work with them is to restore the functioning, resolve the inner conflicts, and solve the tasks of adult living. We speak primarily about adults who have, to a large degree, achieved maturity.

The adolescent comes to us not only with illness, emotional distress, and symptoms but also with a developmental problem. The patient and the therapist must cope with the growing-up process as well as the illness. Blos (1962) speaks of the phase of adolescence as that of the second individuation. The first individuation takes place in early childhood and establishes the psychological self and object, the first separation in terms of the experience of self, while the second individuation deals with separation on a higher level, another phase of the individuation-separation process. Erikson (1950) speaks of the task of adolescence as one of establishing a higher form of identity, of using the identity moratorium to prepare to separate from the family unit, to find a work purpose in life, and to find new and higher forms of intimacy. It is during that time of individuation, of identity formation, of separation and struggle with adult intimacy, that the adolescent comes to us. The adolescent is overwhelmed by the new tasks—to move out of the parental home, find gratification in friendship and love, and progress toward economic independence. Freud (1913) suggested that mental health consists of the capacity to work and to love. It is interesting to try to define the specific phases of that capacity, to work and to love, as they evolve from infancy to adulthood.

The child at puberty, the young adolescent, or the older adolescent moving toward adulthood usually comes to us for treatment when this capacity to work and to love is in jeopardy, endangered by the additional tasks the young person has to meet in our culture, namely, beginning to separate from the parental home; forming an identity; forming new, intimate relationships; and establishing fidelity. One of the characteristics of these young people is either overt or covert rebellion in the home or school or social withdrawal. Such withdrawal patterns indirectly express covert rebellion and overt helplessness, a lack of capacity to meet the world, to slowly let go of the parental home, and to try to resolve the conflicts hindering the task of growing up. Many of our borderline adolescents, as well as those who cope with psychotic illness and mental breakdown, show magnified pictures of the pathological response to separation.

It is at this time that the adolescent comes for help, often unwillingly, coached or forced by parents and teachers. He has to start psychotherapy by trying to begin the treatment, to become attached to the therapeutic situation, to evolve a relationship with the therapist, when actually his major task is separation. *Attachment* behavior and *separation* behavior, about which Bowlby (1969, 1973, 1980) taught us so much, are now in acute conflict. The adolescent must develop a new attachment to the therapist at the same time he is supposed to cope with the task of separation, of creating some form of independence, of developing adult autonomy and the capacity for self-maintenance.

A clinical vignette from the beginning of an adolescent's treatment pictures the struggle between the search for new attachment and the move toward a new self. The patient's reaching out for the therapist, his struggle against him while he searches for a new, reliable object, is also a search for a new, reliable self but is dominated by self and object pathology. The patient, whom I had seen a number of years before (Ekstein 1980a), had called for an appointment. During puberty, he had been referred to another child analyst, but he did not continue treatment very long and became a child at risk. There were episodes of running away, involvement in the drug culture (including selling drugs), and finally return to the parents who had originally sent him to me. This time, he told me, he was really ready for treatment, in contrast to the first time when he interrupted the treatment because he had been sent by the parents. Now he wanted to take responsibility for his own actions, for initiating the treatment. I was able to offer two or three months for a treatment program. He wanted to have one more independent vacation and travel to Afghanistan. He had taken such trips before, and he actually thought it would help him.

I wondered whether some of his friends had been in Afghanistan. Did he play with the idea that he could bring things back from Afghanistan, perhaps drugs, and did they tell him about the risks? Yes, indeed he did know about Afghanistan prisons and the danger. I then wondered why he was more afraid of me, of starting psychotherapy with me, than he was of prisons in Afghanistan. He was puzzled, smiled in embarrassment, and was ready to start the very next day.

The fear of psychotherapy, the fear of the object, and the fear of the discovery of the pathological self was for one moment much stronger than the wish for the emergence of a new self. The new self was to face a dangerous world; to explore it; and to deal with distant, dangerous persecutors in that world. His view of the adult world was well characterized through the journey that he wanted to make, a journey into uncertainty and danger, in which he would have been supported only by his pathological self.

The wish for the analyst's protection, the regression to the kind of helplessness that such a program would initiate, was in conflict with the pathological progression characterized through the fantasy of the flower child, a fantasy that he not only dreamed about but wanted to act out. One might think of this struggle as one between the dependent and independent self, an unhappy and almost impossible choice in view of the patient's background, the family and peers who made up his social environment. I have played with the question, Could the way of beginning be in some form also the way of ending? The ending with such patients frequently will be as unreliable, uncertain, and un- predictable as the beginning. The separation process might be one in which the safe therapeutic alliance is to be exchanged for the adventure of independence, an adventure in which the graduate must play, in fan- tasy or in acting out, with the Afghanistans of the world. As the adoles- cents are about to terminate treatment, cross the bridge toward separation and adulthood and face an uncertain future, they create countertransferences in us. As we now trust their new self, it may make us wish to hold on to the safer territory with which we want them to be connected. Thus attachment and separation are problems not only for the patient but for the therapist as well.

During the phase of the first individuation, the small child ac- complishes the nightly separation from the mother by sustaining him- self psychologically with a "transitional object" (Winnicott 1953). By this means the child can relinquish the mother for the night and transfer his attachment to the transitional object, the teddy bear or blanket. In doing so he slowly gives up the infantile tie to the parental love object and replaces it with a maturer bond rather than helpless bondage.

One might say that the adolescent in conflict now has the task of finding transitional objects, the teddy bears of adolescence, in order to be able to leave home. We think of many youth organizations (social or asocial as we may judge them), of cults, of religious organizations, of youth leaders, of admired school teachers, and so on, which serve as such replacements. The culturally available transitional objects help the adolescent in many of the growth processes to accomplish the slow process of separation from the parental home and later help the adoles- cent reestablish an adult relationship with parents.

In treating adolescents, the significance of the attachment to the therapist is doubled since it is the vehicle to aid the most suitable separation from the home. The subsequent separation from the psychotherapist during termination should lead the adolescent to a higher form of the capacity to attach himself to other people, for example, parents, peers, lovers, employers, and teachers. This reversal of the therapeutic situation gives the therapist a special task as he comes to the end phase of psychotherapy.

In many ways the end phase will be a mirror image of the beginning phase. The question must be raised, Can there be true termination of treatment in the sense that one achieves a previously defined goal? Most people who work with adolescents know that a good many of the treatments seem to end in failure. Interruptions are a kind of termination, not really agreed on by both therapist and the young person because they have reached a goal, but a termination by withdrawal on the part of the adolescent who often breaks up the treatment, does not want to come any longer, and fights against the therapist in the same way he rebels at home and school.

The word "rebellion" is, of course, to be understood primarily as a descriptive label, perhaps an unnecessarily condemning label, because we will understand the rebellion only if we withhold value judgment and think of the adolescent rebellion as a psychic task undertaken to bring about the capacity for separation, even though the breaking up of the early attachment is subjectively experienced by young and old as a rebellion against the adult world. It is usually seen by the parents and by society at large as an unwelcome, defiant rejection of adult morality and culture, while it is viewed by the young person as the search for new and better moral values or as a rejection of the bad of adult society.

Rebellion, however, often turns into helpless submission, endless withdrawal, lack of capacity to communicate, and a search for solutions in loneliness and isolation; or it becomes a negative rebellion which looks like total passivity and total breakdown of mental functioning.

The beginning of treatment frequently depends on the psychotherapist's capacity to win the young patient over, to click with him, a capacity which not many therapists possess, which can hardly be taught, and which may fluctuate from case to case. With some patients I could "click" and with other patients I could not, and the latter I lost quickly. If, however, one can win over such patients, they view the therapist as allied with them in the struggle against parents, school, and society—as one who understands. Such therapists are experienced by the adolescent as secret collaborators, transitional parents, so to speak, who are better than the real parents and who are constantly challenged by adolescents to join them in the struggle. The alliance is,

129

of course, a shaky one. The psychotherapist depends on the parents as well and has to find some way to work with them and see their point of view. If he overidentifies with the adolescent he may turn the parents against his work, and vice versa.

During the end phase the adolescent may frequently behave as he did vis-à-vis the parents. He will try to break up the treatment, declare himself well much earlier than may be the case, and escape into pseudohealth. The therapist often faces the danger of behaving like a parent and holding on to the patient who, he thinks, is not yet ready to separate since the work is not yet finished. These transference and countertransference conditions are closely connected with the developmental task, the necessity to move toward autonomy and independence, albeit through the use of the therapist. The therapist, as transitional object-parent substitute, also must learn to let go but cannot always measure correctly when he should let go as he shifts back and forth in trial identification with the worlds of the adolescent and of the adult.

It is because of this psychological dilemma that a good many cases are terminated although treatment has led to no permanent success. These become repetitions of earlier educational or therapeutic failures. Many cases give us the impression that they were merely interrupted and should have been continued later. One could say that some cases were interrupted with a mutual understanding between therapist and patient. The patient may have wanted to come back later or may have wanted to consult another therapist. One could speak of these patients, to use the words of Margaret Mahler,[1] as going through intermittent treatment.

The therapist must be flexible during the end phase, which is often imposed on him and is experienced by him as the breaking up of treatment, an interruption of treatment, a failure. That may be true in many cases, but in some cases he may overreact instead of responding to the patient's needs.

Generally, we might say that the treatment could end if the responses of the patient to life situations, school, work, and relationships with peers and with parents have again assumed normal proportions. But these normal proportions come about when the developmental task is not yet finished. What is true of children in treatment is true of adolescents: there is still dependence on the parents for economic and emotional support; there is unfinished business in school and work preparation; and there are unstable and changing relationships in friendships and beginning and experimental love situations.

These problems are enhanced through an unstable culture, unstable parental homes, a high divorce rate, unstable economic opportunities, and a youth culture which is much more complex than those of previous generations. Shifting political and religious beliefs and social values, the drug culture, the overabundance in our consumer society: all these very frequently create an environment for the adolescent which makes his own behavior, his own problems, almost society syntonic. Is our society adolescent? Is the adolescent therefore an adult? In such circumstances, how are we to measure the mental health of the adolescent as we move toward the end of treatment?

Can we be psychotherapists who are willing to let the adolescent go but in such a way that our concern for him, our interest in him, is now internalized in him so that he can return after a good experience?

These issues are magnified when we deal with the termination of treatment with adolescents who suffer from severe borderline and psychotic conditions. Can there be an end with such cases? With some we know that endless treatment, or the endless availability of treatment, might be necessary. End of treatment, then, is not an end but, rather, insurance of the ability to maintain a professional or social relationship which allows the patient to return from time to time. It is as if such patients cannot achieve stable, lasting identifications with the therapist (thus having a built-in transitional object, or an eternal inner representation of the object, i.e., an eternal internalized teddy bear) but instead have unstable identifications that have to be periodically restored. In other words, whenever the teddy bear is lost, it has to be established through another phase of treatment.

In an earlier article (1973) on termination process with psychotic adolescents, I referred to the myth of Hercules struggling with the giant who must touch Mother Earth again in order to have his strength grow anew so that he can continue the struggle. The psychotherapist here would be a kind of Hercules who does not prevent the adolescent (the giant) from touching Mother Earth again but, rather, gives him the opportunity to touch Mother Earth from time to time, that is, to touch the therapist to replenish his strength and start anew. Instead of Mother Earth he will have a substitute father or substitute mother therapist.

It is true for all of psychotherapy that we accompany our patients during an important phase of their lives. Termination is not only their problem but ours as well. This is doubly true in the treatment of adolescents. A part in us feels about them as if they were our own children. We cope with our own problem of letting go. The countertransference feelings, as one gets attached to the psychotherapeutic task, can be compared to vibrations as they take place in the parents who do not know whether they have fulfilled their parental functioning, who need their children in their own way, in fulfilling their own lives, and so on. Fulfilling professional obligations presents a special problem for those who work with adolescents, whose very natural inclination is to cope with separation as if it were a violent process. How difficult it is for them and for us to learn from a comment that Freud once made to Theodor Reik (1949) when Reik found it difficult to say good-bye to him, thinking they might not see each other again. Freud said, "People who belong together do not need to stay glued together." The uncertainty about the outcome, and the uncertainty of the adolescent's future, makes it hard for us to let go. We want to be sure we have done enough for him and with him.

Earlier conceptions of the outcome of the analytic process, conceptions that we learned from the pioneers, at times made us idealize the end of the treatment. We thought that when the repressed trauma is brought to consciousness it is dissolved, and the patient is enabled to fulfill his growth process and move toward self-realization, free of the pain of the past. Erikson (1950) once spoke, half seriously and half in jest, about the myth of the psychoanalytic man. The cure was to achieve postambivalent heterosexuality. Each society, he suggested, creates its own myth of perfection, whether it is the ideal Christian society and the Christian man, a communist society and the true communist man serving the state, a capitalist society and the true individualistic man, or the psychoanalytic world of perfect cure. Such early idealizations have to be given up. Therapeutic processes do not completely overcome residual trauma, a concept stressed by Blos (1962).

I will now illustrate some of the multifaceted issues in the process of termination utilizing early material from the research records of a patient referred to as Elaine (Ekstein 1955, 1956, 1961). This case will remind us of some of the difficulties of psychotherapy research with patients whose treatment spans a long period of time and for whom a comparatively long period is necessary for adequate follow-up studies. However, this can also result in a diminishing reliability of information since both memory and electronic tapes fade with the years.

Termination must not be considered an arbitrary point in the treatment curve; rather, it is a process in itself (Ekstein 1965, 1973). It is a unique part of the treatment, just as the diagnostic process and the opening gambit are. The issues paramount in the end phase are those of separation, mourning, giving up the love object, the working through of the total process; a kind of epilogue which is a prologue for the future, an after play which restates what has been said before. But it is now said in the language dictated by a stronger ego more capable of utilizing synthetic and integrative functions in the service of secondary process functioning. Now we deal with stronger self and object relations. The inner dialogue must have moved away from fluctuating self and object representations toward a more stable sense of self as well as stable objects and a more stable internal representation of the significant people in the patient's life.

We are interested in discovering whether the end phases with psychotics and borderlines are different from those of neurotics and in what ways they differ. Federn (1952) stated that there can be no termination with psychotics, and one must continue some kind of professional or social relationship which will encourage the patient to return occasionally if the need recurs. Such a philosophy implies that the transference cannot and should not be dissolved because of the patient's inability to make stable identifications. This results in his only being able to maintain the introject of the analyst, revived and/or strengthened in the patient by the presence of the therapist, to replenish the internal representation, thus allowing also for the replenishing of the self. Heinrich Heine (1844), speaking of his secret return to Germany while living in exile in France, referred to himself as the giant who had touched Mother Earth again, thus having his strength grow anew.

How are we to assess a termination philosophy which seems to be in the nature of a self-fulfilling prophecy as a necessary postulate for treating adolescents? We have assumed that this process can have a termination phase.

Case 1

In the following illustration a true termination phase seemed possible while the therapist remained alive in the patient's mind after many years, with each having maintained peripheral contact with the other.

Elaine, a thirteen-year-old, was brought to treatment against her will following a 2,000-mile summer vacation trip with her mother. She did not know that the trip would end at the Menninger Clinic rather than at Niagara Falls. She insisted on going to Niagara Falls where she wanted to experience a delusional honeymoon with Robin Hood, a delusional love object whom she was to wed. This delusional love object was the only inner support she had to feed a starved self. The nature of this delusion was such that it was presented at times as a fantasy and at other times as a true psychotic delusional system leading to suicidal and homicidal attempts during the more acute phases of the illness. At still other times the delusion was under sufficient control so that a full and open break with reality was avoided, thus leading to the diagnosis of borderline schizophrenia. I have since wondered whether today we might not diagnose her as a borderline.

Elaine was a deeply religious girl whose convictions became part of a system of communication with the therapist with whom she was not able to identify completely but would "devour" in the beginning phases of her therapy. This was typical of all her relationshps, which were dominated by the pull toward fusion states in which she became the love object with whom she wanted to identify. Thus, she could only become Christ rather than Christlike, which was her stated ego ideal. Elaine was seen three times per week for four years and achieved a fairly complete recovery. She progressed from the hospital to a boarding home, to high school, and later to a boarding college.

The following material describes some of the end phase of Elaine's treatment during a time when she was anticipating a very successful graduation from high school. She had to choose between attending a nearby university, which would enable her to continue treatment, and attending another institution out of the area, which would necessitate ending treatment.

In this interview, she speaks about the anticipated complete or partial separation in a few months. The interview is taken directly from the tape and is essentially one in which we deal with transference and countertransference issues. If one were listening to the material, one would be impressed by the normal-sounding nature of the girl's responses but would also be reminded of the "cobra's egg" in which the young cobra can be seen. In the egg, the dangerous cobra is perfectly formed but covered by a transparent membrane.

THERAPIST: How are you?
PATIENT: Okay.

THERAPIST: When I walked out a minute ago I thought you were completely . . . how do you call that?

PATIENT: Absorbed?

THERAPIST: Absorbed in yourself, and you started a review of literature or whatever you read. You didn't even notice that I walked by. But I suspected you knew. Did you have some inkling I walked by?

PATIENT: You spoke to me, didn't you?

THERAPIST: I know. But you sort of, well, I guess you didn't hear me.

PATIENT: I guess you whispered.

THERAPIST: Is that a new sweater?

PATIENT: No.

THERAPIST: Can't remember seeing it.

PATIENT: It's a little difficult to wear this sweater because it is so low-necked. So I wear another sweater with it. You may have seen it, but generally I wear it on days like this. I think it looks really dressy that way.

THERAPIST: Nice.

PATIENT: It isn't too low-necked when I wear it like this. But the way it is now it is dramatic on me.

THERAPIST: It does look very sharp.

PATIENT: How do you mean? Okay?

THERAPIST: Okay. No pressures of life impinging on you?

PATIENT: Quite a few.

THERAPIST: You don't sound like they are emergencies.

PATIENT: One of them has me very much upset. You know the kids I run around with, Marcia, Maxie, you know they . . .

THERAPIST: You mentioned that, uh.

PATIENT: Well this all started last summer when, well you know. It's pretty rowdy. And we've been trying for a long time to get a leader. And last Sunday night these folks came to our meeting. And by the time they came we had evolved to the point where we were singing hymns with her, that teacher. And then we went downstairs and we tried to play Ping-Pong. Then we played for a while and were noisy, and then the boys decided to play one more game, and Marcia, Vickie, and I decided to cheer for them, and so we named them real odd names—"this-and-that," or "thing-a ma-bob," something like that. Then they changed courts and went over to the other side, you know, not courts, but whatever you call it, Ping-Pong courts. They went to the other side to a table anyway. And so we decided to change their names. Well, somebody suggested "Brown Noses."

THERAPIST: I'm sorry. What did you say?

PATIENT: Brown noses. Brownies.

THERAPIST: Brownies. Cookies or Girl Scouts?

PATIENT: People who polish apples.

THERAPIST: They're called brown noses? Brownies? I never heard that before.

PATIENT: Or, they get Brownie points.

THERAPIST: Oh, is that the same little Brownies who work for little points? No, I don't know what it is anyway.

PATIENT: Well, anyway, they polish apples. You call one group Brownies and Brown Noses. Well, we were trying to think of names you know. Somebody suggested Brown Noses and they said no, that two syllables were better instead of one or three. So I said all right, why don't we have Brownies, and Marcia popped up with the "Fairies." I mean I think I suggested before that we have the odds and the queens. But I was just kidding. And we laughed louder and so we started out cheering, you know.

THERAPIST: The Brown Noses and the Fairies.

PATIENT: They started cheering and I started cheering for them in church. These people in church, these people who were trying to make an impression on . . . and we cheered all the way through now. Well, I did too, but not too much.

As one attempts to make sense of the metaphoric language of the therapeutic dialogue, one can see that the stage is set very early in this hour by the discussion of the two sweaters, the two ego or self organizations which she brings to treatment and how she speaks metaphorically of the precarious adjustments that she has achieved between the fluctuating states of shifting selves and objects. Such a conflict is a constant problem in all her object relationships where she seems to be torn between sexual desires and her pseudoreligious convictions, or sexual identifications, male or female. Unstable object relations are hinted at constantly throughout the hour, although she masters them or covers them with a veneer of adjustment. She gives her version of the adolescent conflict when she introduces the issue about who the queens and the odds are. In this way, through references to these external representations, she brings to us her observations and reflections about herself while the therapist attempts to translate them back into direct observations about herself. That is, he attempts to restore the synthetic functioning in order that these issues are not split off once more from the rest of the personality.

During this session, as she speaks of her conflicts with her peers from her religious group, we are reminded of earlier representations of the internal images—the Christ to whom she used to pray (Ekstein 1956) and with whom she fused and King David who is to press Bathsheba (Ekstein 1961)—and of her move away from the more primitive preoccupation with the Bible and her own development toward the current normal adolescent peer group.

Then our patient tells us of her difficulties in church—God does not appear through the open door as she expected Him to—and we are actually hearing a description of the loss of the secondary gains of the psychotic experience. We realize that she is telling us how the treatment has taken previously available psychotic resources away from her. Quasi-religious, delusional experience can still be wished for, hoped for, but now she must mourn the loss of the psychosis, just as we mourn the loss of childhood with its magic and wonderland, which is also a period of unstable ego organization and shifting self- and object-representations. She reminds one of the Space Child (Wright and Ekstein 1964) who told his therapist that he would always blame her for taking away his enjoyable space fantasies—even though she did not forbid them, she took them away by curing him to the point that his reality testing grew and his capacity to lose himself in such fantasies was gone. We also hear the patient tell us that she wants to return in the future, in the way that people who have been hospitalized for a lengthy time might want to return frequently to the ward with a faint nostalgia even though the ward was the place of their suffering. We are reminded of comments made earlier (Ekstein 1965) which describe the termination period as the after play, a form of thanksgiving which the patient celebrates with, and for, the therapist. We hear the therapist restating to his patient the gains that she has achieved in treatment, particularly with regard to the fact that if she ever needs help again she will be able to come on her own rather than having to be forced into treatment.

COMMENT

At the end of treatment we usually expect, throughout the process of termination, that the symptomatology has disappeared, that the synthetic capacity of the ego, which would permit integration of impulse life with the life of reality and with the dictates of the conscience, has been restored. In other words, we expect a resolution of internal and, to some extent, external conflict. We expect that the patient's mental life will be dominated by a restored capacity for reality testing in order to maintain a balance between the involvement with inner fantasy life and with external reality. We have seen how reality testing is linked with the capacity for object relations, and we expect, at the termination of treatment, a visible development of a mature capacity for object relations accompanied by a mature concept of the self. We expect that the individual is now capable of putting thought before act rather than immediately discharging an impulse, acting out, and rationalizing post hoc. We expect that the dominance of the symbolic function of language has been restored and that speech no longer serves merely as a signal or as a trigger but is now dominated by the secondary process and the functioning of symbolic communication. At the end of treatment, we expect that the individual will continue to *dream,* but now in the service of the waking process in order to realize the future, rather than merely falling back on the past.

Comparatively few complete cases have been reported in the literature which actually describe the termination process in the treatment of psychotic children. If the goals above were actually achieved in the treatment of a psychotic child or adolescent patient, we would expect to see a psychic organization somewhat similar to that of the neurotic patient. The main difference would be with respect to the psychic organization at the beginning of treatment. However, in the treatment of the psychotic patient we do not find an ending picture similar to that of the neurotic one. Nor do we find the same kind of progression along the various dimensions conceptualized in our view of the treatment process. The very differences that exist at the onset of treatment dictate a different course in the treatment process. In the psychotic child or adolescent most of the deficit is seen in the area of ego development. Therefore, we usually begin to deal with a psychotic organization in which there is a powerful disequilibrium with a tendency toward regressive functioning. This in itself creates an unbalanced position during the psychotherapeutic process, somewhat like a pendulum that moves with a larger arc to the left than to the right. Thus, we find that the overt symptomatology which brings the patient, or, more accurately, drives the patient, to seek treatment seems to be more pronounced with the psychotic patient and is more frightening to the adult world. This symptomatology invites a different kind of handling than would be true for the neurotic child. Thus, we often find a deep hate and enormous anxiety in the parents that cannot be mastered by them and is very often also found in other people in the patient's environment who have been provoked by the patient. School personnel, peers, and even clinic personnel are subject to similar reactions which are disguised by endless waiting lists and lack of resources but are actually due in part to the situation of the professional staff who are frightened by the involvement and commitment necessary to treat such patients. It is also true of the social response of the entire community and government agencies in the funding of such clinics. It is truly an almost impossible feat to create a treatment situation which can be maintained and supported by the community and therapist, who often find it difficult to cope with the inevitable nightmare-like features characteristic of such patients before, or even while in, therapy. These children can be treated only by acknowledging the impossible nature of the feat—while denying it at the same time.

It is the regressive curve during the treatment that is in full swing. That regressive curve can be found not only in the area of instinctual regression but also in the area of ego regression, or, more aptly, in the area of ego fixations at lower levels of organization. These fixations are frequently of a kind that tempts us to say that we deal here with an organic deficit beyond repair, and thus we acquire a rationale (or is it a rationalization?) to avoid any involvement in a psychotherapeutic program.

The nature of the progressive curve differs from that in the treatment of a neurotic child inasmuch as we now deal with autistic imitations of, rather than true identifications with, the therapist. Often we find that what looks like progressive movement in the ego is merely a facade, resembling the impostor who pretends to be something that he is not, that he really cannot be.

As we look at the transference development we find even greater differences, even though we can recognize some neurotic and pseudoneurotic manifestations in cases with children and adolescents. However, it is the psychotic transference features that make it necessary for us to remodel our basic assumptions of the treatment process. Ordinarily, we can rely on a strong observing, reflecting ego organization which offers an ally in the treatment process. With the psychotic patient we find the ego is either nonexistent or fluctuates and operates only in the presence of the therapist, like the impostor (Abraham 1935) or the as-if personality (Deutsch 1934), whose chameleon-like qualities result in an incapacity to maintain any achieved change under different conditions or circumstances. Since we cannot rely on the observing, reflecting functions of the ego as an ally, we must find new ones. With the psychotic patient we must ally ourselves with the delusional features. These are all we have to work with because they are the elements which are most dominant in the personality. Since we must work with weak, dangerous, and unreliable allies, with delusional monsters and creatures (whom we hope we can slowly influence by accepting them as allies), we must recognize the danger inherent in such "reactionary" regressive helpers. Their strength is derived from the fact that they are more real and valid to the patient than the superficial facade of imitative ego functioning. Thus, the psychotic transference leads to immense technical difficulties for the therapist.

The peculiar nature of the psychotic transferences is paralleled by an extraordinary countertransference potential, with both positive and negative aspects, which can, when utilized, lead to successful treatment or to interruptions and disruptions. For example, the usual analytic stance of freely suspended attention is unavailable in work with such children and adolescents since it cannot be matched in the patient by the capacity to observe and to clarify. The therapist's own unconscious is drawn into the psychotic process, and he is threatened with immense anxiety in which his only defense is to struggle, to avoid the delusional material. Frequently, he can do this only by becoming an educator in order to avoid his own unconscious and his own psychotic potential. It is as if he must escape from the wonderland into the living room, to run away from Alice rather than follow her. This may lead to attempts to confront the patient with reality, educate him, adjust him, and hence avoid the resolution of the inner struggle since the inner struggle deals with the primary process. Behavior modification in such cases will not lead us into the wonderland and does push Alice to return to the living room. But she must finish her dream, accompanied by us, where she can gain from the dream and return accompanied, but not pushed, by the therapist.

This countertransference difficulty has been described by one of my patients quite well, as we can see in his response to the Thematic Apperception Test card usually responded to as illustrative of the treatment situation (Ekstein and Caruth 1965): "Hypnotist hypnotizes a subject. Subject is sleeping. Sure enough, subject does everything he says. Subject is asleep. Hypnotist says, 'Repeat after me everything I say.' Subject has to do it. Hypnotist walks away and leaves subject there and hypnotist gets ready for the next thing. This is not a stage. He looks in mirror and practices and puts himself into sleep. Subject wakes up and says, 'Ready for the show,' and the hypnotist says, 'I am asleep, asleep, asleep.' The Hypnotized Hypnotist.''

We see the power of the patient who tries to draw the therapist into his own primary process psychotic fantasy, although in this instance the therapist who had fallen asleep for a moment can interpret and help the patient restore the patient's reflecting ego functions. However, usually when the therapist uses freely suspended attention, he may be pulled into the material too much and may need to ward it off by the well-described countermeasures.

The psychotic transferences which make the therapist into a rescuing god or a helpless puppet are often matched by the impotence and helplessness of the therapist whose megalomania is shattered by the ineffectiveness of his usual tools. Thus, the therapist may fuse with the megalomanic hopes as well as the infantile helplessness of the patient. Here, too, he must struggle against the desire to merge with the patient. How can one maintain a treatment situation without becoming en-meshed in parental environmental functions? Indeed, we need the parents to help. Yet he who depends on parents must remember that "he who pays the piper calls the tune," and the tune of the parents is always "learning, adjustment, growing up," whereas the therapist's task is interpretation and understanding of the unconscious conflict.

Elaine finished her treatment after more than four years. She specialized in literature and became a college teacher. She also remains deeply involved with the church. Later she did practical work with computers and thus combined features of her father (a computer expert) and her grandfather (a minister). She has maintained herself for many years, and occasionally a Christmas card comes my way, which I answer. She has traveled abroad and has seen the Holy Land and the birthplaces of Greco-Judaic culture. It has been about twenty-five years since I have seen her, and I have only occasionally heard from her. Her life is an unusual one, full of competence and creativity but certainly not conventional. Her treatment can be judged as having had a successful outcome even though she does not measure up to certain conventional notions of mental health. Measuring her "capacity to love and to work" requires a redefinition of work and love. But in her own way she is stable, productive, and contributing to society.

Did I let her go too early? Could I have done more? These questions lead me to another vignette of the end phase in the treatment of another adolescent. This vignette illustrates the questions that arise in the mind of the therapist and patient about whether they can let go of each other; whether the residual trauma is no more than a weak reminder of the past and will not lead to new regressions, as the patient faces the task of moving toward independence and establishing more mature self and object relationships.

Case 2

The boy, age fifteen, started his treatment under emergency conditions (Ekstein 1980b). This high schooler's father was absent; he lived with his mother and sister. He was to meet the therapist because of stealing episodes and unmanageable behavior at home. The night before, he and friends broke into their high school, stole musical instruments, and were arrested. He came directly from the police station to the therapist. He entered anxiously, slowly telling about the events. The therapist wondered why the patient had not come before the break-in. The boy admitted he should have done that, reading the comment of the therapist as reproach. The therapist, recalling the techniques of Aichhorn (1925), told him that the way they went about stealing was incompetent. If he had come earlier, perhaps the therapist could have told him how to steal with success. The boy, in response to whether he was competent otherwise, said that he was an excellent vaulter on the school's gymnastics team. He looked at a picture that the therapist had under glass on his desk, a photograph of his own son winning an athletic competition and getting a medal. Wouldn't he, the patient, rather get a gold medal than find himself in jail, losing school privileges, and so forth? A therapeutic alliance was established. The therapist had identified himself, so to speak, with the unsuccessful thief, telling him that he could have taught him how to be a successful thief. The boy, identifying himself with the therapist's son, aimed at the gold medal.

Slowly, this patient permitted the therapist to enter his inner world. The boy watched his favorite television show, the goings-on in the spaceship, a mission impossible. In fantasy he fell in love with a young woman clerk on that spaceship. Over succeeding weeks he developed a theme, a quasi-autobiographical fantasy with himself as the hero of the space adventure. Actually, he played two heroes, his split selves. He

142

became the captain of the spaceship, and he was also one of the musicians, a nightclub singer. In his fantasy, both men dance with the fantasy lady in question. The captain was described as someone who knew engineering and techniques of space technology (reminiscent of a goal that his father had in mind for the boy, hoping that his son would become an engineer), but he also played the part of a musician (an ideal of the Hollywood world that was much nearer to the fantasy expectations of his mother). He was involved in an endless struggle between allegiance to the mother and hope for alliance with the father. Under what conditions, then, would the young woman love him? Should he be the captain or should he be the musician? Only slowly did he dare to risk himself, and he finally confessed to her that he was both. He was ready now to search for a new self, an integrated self, and saw himself moving through high school, being successful in athletics, going on with music, trying to find a music group, and preparing himself for college. Thus he would not only meet the aspirations of both parents but also heal the split in himself, the disparate, painful psychic injury, reinforced through the prolonged and traumatic divorce struggle of the parents.

He saw himself accepted by the therapist, who had discovered long before that the young fantasy woman of the spaceship was no more than a transitional object, the adolescent teddy bear (Winnicott 1953).

As treatment moved toward ending he found employment, a wish of his father's, but in a music store. This was a dream he had not given up as he moved toward graduation and achieved the gold medal. At the same time, he became involved in some drug activities, being fearful of separation from the therapist, since he would have to move out of the community for college and be exposed to an uncertain and unsafe peer culture.

In the working through of his fantasy he had written a new script, got his act together, so to speak, and restored the different fragments of self to a total self. Will the restoration hold? Will the self fall apart again? Will old traumata, the residual traumata, bring about new regression?

As he leaves the therapy, the *Spielraum*, the play space, will change, and the demands will be harsher.

I concluded the description of this case as follows (Ekstein 1980):

Ending the psychotherapy is a trauma, a sad and an anxiety-arousing event. If it is a growth trauma it will lead to genuine individuation. If it came prematurely it might bring on new regression. The positive trauma of the therapeutic experience, the belief of the therapist in the patient's capacity to win the gold medal, that reversal of rejection and punishment, of anger and parental rage, has traumatic impact on the patient insofar as it destroys the acquired position of the delinquent facade and fosters the withdrawal, the inner preoccupation with self. How is one to measure the permanency of change? What is the boundary line that will either allow the residual trauma to remain primarily a move towards growth or develop in regressive terms? This boy, it seems, has a second chance.

As a young adult experiencing stress, trying to get a perspective on the uncertain times just before the Second World War, I identified myself with Thomas Mann's hero Hans Castorp. I lost myself in the story of his life in the days when my native Austria was invaded. Thomas Mann, ending his novel *The Magic Mountain* (1924), tells about Hans Castorp, who spent a long time in a sanitorium in order to recover from tuberculosis and, perhaps, severe emotional problems and found himself in an in-between situation almost like that of an adolescent in treatment. In the last few pages Thomas Mann describes Hans Castorp as he leaves treatment and the Magic Mountain. We slowly lose sight of him. In the last view we have of Hans Castorp, he is in the army at the beginning of the First World War. Ordered to regain the position the enemy had taken the day before, Hans and the other young men storm the enemy lines at dawn. Comrades fall. He grits his teeth and races on. Fog sometimes makes it impossible for him to see, and we, too, cannot see him. Finally he disappears, and we do not know what will happen to him. Will he meet the tasks of life, the encounters with love and hate, or will he falter? As he runs we hear him humming a beautiful poem about words of love he wants to carve into the bark of trees as everlasting proof of his yearning for love and his preparedness for love. We no longer see what will happen to him. Will there be a successful adult life for him? Or will he end as flotsam? Will he survive the gathering storm?

When I spoke about termination of psychoanalysis of adults I preceded that essay with the words of Shakespeare, "The past is prologue," but as one ends treatment with adolescents one can say only that treatment is perhaps the prologue of the future. The ending of treatment is but the beginning of a new life.

In work with adults, we restore somewhat normal functioning. In work with adolescents, we clear the way for further development, but we cannot predict where it is going to lead. Withstanding this pain of uncertainty, often disguised as a scientific dilemma, is a capacity the therapist must acquire in order to cope with adolescence, with adolescent patients who revive in him the uncertainty of his own adolescence.

By chance I was able to maintain contact with some former patients, with whom I started treatment during their puberty or adolescence, and I learned much later that I was used by them toward a better future. One recalls then that it is not the therapist who changes patients, but, rather, it is the patient who uses the therapist to change his life. Omnipotence then gives way to omnipotentiality, a form of uncertainty, a task to be solved rather than a fantasy by which to be plagued.

NOTES

1. Personal communication with M. Mahler, 1966.

REFERENCES

Abraham, K. 1935. The history of an impostor in the light of psychoanalytic knowledge. *Psychoanalytic Quarterly* 4:570–587.

Aichhorn, A. 1925. *Verwonderluste Jugend* [Wayward youth]. Leipzig: Psychoanalytischer.

Blos, P. 1962. *On Adolescence*. Glencoe, Ill.: Free Press.

Bowlby, J. 1969, 1973, 1980. *Attachment and Loss*. Vols. 1–3. New York: Basic.

Deutsch, H. 1934. On a type of pseudo-affectivity—the "as if." *Internationale Zeitschrift für Arztliche Psychoanalyse* 20:323–335.

Ekstein, R. 1955. Vicissitudes of the "internal image" in the recovery of a borderline schizophrenic adolescent. *Bulletin of the Menninger Clinic* 29:86–92.

Ekstein, R. 1956. A clinical note on the therapeutic use of a quasi-religious experience. *Journal of the American Psychoanalytic Association* 4:304–313.

Ekstein, R. 1961. Cross-sectional views in the psychotherapeutic process with an adolescent girl recovering from a schizophrenic episode. *American Journal of Orthopsychiatry* 31:757–775.

Ekstein, R. 1965. Working through and termination of analysis. *Journal of the American Psychoanalytic Association* 13:57–58.

Ekstein, R. 1973. The process of termination and its relation to outcome in the treatment of psychotic disorders in adolescence. *Adolescent Psychiatry* 3:448–460.

Ekstein, R. 1980a. Borderline states and ego disturbances. In G. Sholevar, M. Benson, and B. Blinder, eds. *Treatment of Emotional Disorders in Children and Adolescents*. New York: Spectrum.

Ekstein, R. 1980b. Residual trauma—variation on and about a theme. *Family and Child Mental Health Journal* 6:34–62.

Ekstein, R., and Caruth, E. 1965. Working alliance with the monster. *Bulletin of the Menninger Clinic* 29:189–197.

Erikson, E. 1950. *Childhood and Society*. New York: Norton.

Federn, P. 1952. *Ego Psychology and the Psychoses*. New York: Basic.

Freud, S. 1913. On beginning the treatment. Further recommendations on the technique of psychoanalysis. *Standard Edition* 12:121–144. London: Hogarth, 1958.

Heine, H. 1844. *Deutschland, ein Wintermärchen*.

Mann, T. 1924. *Magic Mountain*. New York: Knopf.

Reik. T. 1949. *From 30 Years with Freud*. New York: International Universities Press.

Winnicott, D. 1953. Transitional objects and transitional phenomena. *International Journal of Psychoanalysis* 34:59–97.

Wright, D., and Ekstein, R. 1964. The space child ten years later. *Forest Hospital Publications* 2:36–47.

11   EARLY ADOLESCENT DEAF BOYS:
A BIOPSYCHOSOCIAL APPROACH

CARL B. FEINSTEIN

Introduction

It has long been recognized that psychiatric disorders are a major problem among hearing-impaired and deaf children and adolescents. Previous writings in this area, however, have focused on general considerations regarding the personality traits and psychopathology of deaf children. Much less has been written about deaf adolescents. In particular, there is a paucity of information regarding the *ongoing experience* of deafness and how it affects the emotional development of the deaf adolescent. Moreover, little has been written about how either psychodynamic factors or the many disruptions and distortions in the process of communication influence personality traits and psychopathology in deaf youth.

This chapter will specifically address some important psychosocial, psychodynamic, and neuropsychiatric issues which shape and color the personality development and behavior of deaf adolescents. The diversity of institutions, sociocultural backgrounds, and educational methods which deaf children experience makes it difficult to characterize this entire population. The sample which provided the clinical basis for this paper is weighted toward children from lower-middle-class and indigent households whose educational method emphasized signing and "total communication" in verbal interactions. However, the need for clinical information about deaf adolescents is considerable, and I have elected to describe the findings from my experience, hoping that psychiatrists familiar with different subsets of the deaf population will be stimulated to fill in the gaps or point out the differences.

REVIEW OF THE LITERATURE

Many authors have reported a typical personality constellation for the deaf child which includes the characteristics of rigidity, egocentricity, absence of creativity, lack of empathy, deficits in inner controls, suggestibility, and impulsivity (Altshuler 1971, 1978; Freeman, Malkin, and Hastings 1975; Mindel and McCay 1971; Schlesinger 1977; Vernon 1967; Williams 1970). In a Los Angeles survey of teachers, Schlesinger and Meadow (1972) found the incidence of behavioral problems among deaf children at a residential school to be *31.2 percent*. Jensema and Trybus (1975), in their annual survey of hearing-impaired children in special education programs, reported a 10 percent prevalence of behavioral problems. Schein (1975) reported an 18.9 percent rate for emotional-behavioral problems. Naiman, Schein, and Stewart (1973) found that approximately 10 percent of deaf children are disturbed enough to warrant intervention beyond routine special educational placement. Freeman et al. (1975), in their Vancouver, British Columbia, survey, found an incidence of 22.6 percent of moderate to severe psychiatric disorders. Murphy and Trybus (1975) have reported a high incidence of dropouts from schools for the deaf, and Schein (1975) noted that 10 percent of deaf children eligible for such schools are altogether out of school.

Numerous factors have been cited as contributors to the high incidence of emotional disorder among hearing-impaired children. Studies of children who are deaf because of rubella have reported common behavioral characteristics of restlessness, hyperactivity, distractibility, impulsivity, and instability along with a high incidence of learning disabilities and other neurological sequelae (Chess, Korn, and Fernandez 1971; Desmond, Wilson, Melnick, Singer, Zion, Rudolph, Pineda, Ziai, and Blattner 1967; Schein 1975; Vernon 1967). Chess et al. (1971) found a preponderance of psychiatric symptomatology in their cohort of deaf adolescents with other handicaps secondary to rubella. However, recently Chess and Fernandez (1980) found that the only symptom present more commonly in deaf children without other handicaps when compared with hearing children was "impulsivity."

Delayed language acquisition has been implicated by several authors as a cause of emotional disturbance in deaf children. Lesser and Easser

(1972) hypothesized that this delay leads to problems in the development of secondary process thinking. Galenson, Miller, Kaplan, and Rothstein (1979) asserted that delayed language development distorts the separation-individuation process and leads to problems in the self and object representation. They argued that these distortions result in long-range influences on the personality of the deaf. Stern (1978) cited the deficit in early socialization that he feels is the inevitable concomitant of deprivation of the "music" and emotional content of the vocal interaction between mothers and children. Freedman (1980), however, disagreed with these authors, arguing that myelinization of the CNS pathways relevant to language development occurs mostly after the normal age for negotiation of the separation-individuation process. Rainer (1969), reviewing comparative studies of the psychosocial development of deaf children of deaf parents versus that of deaf children of hearing parents (which indicate better overall adaptation of the former), concluded that "it is the parent-child relationship which is important, rather than the use of verbal speech as such" (Rainer 1976).

For deaf teenagers, the profound disruption of communication and the experiential isolation which result from their condition subject them to unique stresses as they undertake the developmental tasks of adolescence. Regardless of whether the resultant problems are conceptualized theoretically as due to an early distortion of the separation/individuation process or as due to ongoing problems in the parent-child relationship, it is not surprising that these youngsters have trouble negotiating the adolescent phase of development.

However, little is known in depth about psychosocial development in deaf teenagers. Before theory building can progress, before there can be truly meaningful comparisons made between the depth psychology of deaf versus hearing adolescents, we must have a great deal more knowledge, both from a general psychosocial perspective and from the clinical perspective. This chapter is directed toward filling in some of the knowledge gaps which exist concerning the psychosocial realities of being deaf and adolescent.

CLINICAL EXPERIENCE

The clinical experience underlying this presentation was gained by psychiatric consultation to a large special day school for the deaf which emphasizes a "total communications" (signing plus oral speech) approach. The population of this school was skewed toward a more

socioeconomically deprived group and contained an unrepre-
sentatively small number of the most socially advantaged strata for
children. The consultation involved meetings with teachers, supervis-
ory faculty, and counselors, along with frequent classroom observations and direct interviewing of children. For one year, this consultation included a once-weekly psychotherapy group for eight boys aged
thirteen and fourteen attending this school. This group-therapy experience generated several hypotheses regarding the source of some of the
students' behavioral difficulties that were then pursued in other aspects
of the consultation.

Group therapy, or group therapeutic approaches, for deaf youngsters
in the school setting have been previously described by a small number
of authors (Fuhrer and Litoff 1979; Rozek, Sien, Nostoff, and Nower
1979; Sarlin and Altshuler 1968). Many authors have noted the severe
problems these children have in a group setting, whether classroom or
therapeutic. Myklebust (1964) referred to the restricted ability of deaf
children to communicate with each other, resulting in less structured,
more immature, and more "sensory-motor" behaviors. In working
with emotionally disturbed children, Edelstein (1978) found a striking
inability to function on an interpersonal level, especially in group activities. "Many students preferred individual instead of group activities
and in fact did not possess a readiness to function as part of a group."
Naiman and co-workers (1973), in their therapeutic classroom,
established their primary goal as the improvement of social skills and
interpersonal relating, particularly in the group context. In their
therapeutic classroom for deaf adolescents, Rozek and colleagues
(1979) found it necessary to develop special techniques to facilitate
formation of group identification and group interaction among the children. Fuhrer and Litoff (1979), who report on group intervention with
hearing-impaired adolescents in the school setting, described "a larger
amount of visual, verbal and nonverbal interaction in activity occurring
constantly within the group." Sarlin and Altshuler (1968), in their
ground-breaking report of group therapy with deaf adolescents, reported that these adolescents had a "lack of mutual interest" and made
continual efforts to involve the therapist in an exclusive dyadic relationship. They showed little concern for each other and, in general,
demonstrated a high level of activity disruptive to group functioning.

In the group-therapy situation to be described, my cotherapist was a
counselor at the school who not only knew the boys but also had the
somewhat rare ability to interpret and reverse interpret (sign language

or oral speech and reverse) while participating as a cotherapist. The eight boys who participated in this group were selected by the school. All had manifested behavior problems in the school setting, including disruptive and inattentive behavior in and between classes. Several had been in trouble more than once for fighting. However, it should be mentioned that boys with the most serious level of disturbance (severe conduct disorder, psychotic behavior, etc.) were not included in the group.

We found that the boys had serious difficulties interacting with each other in the group setting. Each exhibited an almost continuous yearning to speak at great length about personal experiences at home or school, but every individual's effort to speak at length was met with inattentiveness or outright turning away by the other boys. One factor contributing to this seemed to be a generally short attention span or capacity for "listening" to another's speech. The only boy who seemed slightly more successful at holding the others' attention accomplished this by virtue of his rather remarkable ability to pantomime. There was continuous, fierce competition to speak and to have the visual attention of other boys since, in order to be "listened to," it was necessary to gain the listener's eye contact. The effort to gain eye contact, often by all the boys in the group at once, resulted in endless activity and disruptiveness to the group process. The boys waved hands in each other's faces, jumped up and down, nudged, pushed others' chairs, clowned, hit, and kicked to gain attention. It seemed almost impossible to maintain a single group focus. Instead, the group fragmented into dyads of boys carrying on independent conversations. Aggressive behavior broke out frequently in response to being ignored by others in the group or in response to the efforts of another disruptive boy intent on gaining the group's attention for himself. When the therapist pointed out the difficulty of listening to each other, invariably someone in the group would "side with" the therapist by urging the offending boy to "be cool." This exhortation was always ineffective and frequently led to the exhorter himself becoming frustrated at his inability to gain the listener's attention.

What could possibly explain these overwhelming difficulties? My experience does not support Sarlin and Atshuler's interpretation (1968) that this group behavior represents a "lack of interest" in peers. There were many opportunities to learn about these boys outside the therapy-group setting. Most of them had friends with whom they spent considerable time, generally in groups of two or three, during the very limited times available for this sort of activity in the school. There was a consistent tendency toward social isolation for only one boy in the group and for only a small minority of children in the school. In fact, most of the children this age were now traveling by public transportation to visit each other in the evening and on weekends, further indicating that they were in fact genuinely *interested* in each other and in companionship.

Are these behavioral difficulties in group settings entirely a product of profound underlying deficits in object relations secondary to early language deprivation, or are there more immediate causes? I will focus on three more immediate considerations which I have found to have explanatory value and which indicate possible areas for therapeutic work. These are (1) experiential deprivation in the area of social skills; (2) dynamic considerations centering on low self-esteem, narcissistic vulnerability, and the affect of shame; and (3) formal factors related to communication by sign language in a group setting, including certain possible neuropsychological limiting factors.

SOCIAL FACTORS: EXPERIENTIAL DEPRIVATION AND SOCIAL SKILLS

Furth (1966), in his studies of cognition in the deaf, demonstrated that in most situations poorer performance in cognitive testing of deaf children is not due to some postulated deficit in thinking based on language deficits but, rather, is a result of inadequate experience and information. This experiential deprivation is a direct result of being cut off from all auditory sources of information. Along a similar vein, there is a large body of opinion which asserts that many deaf children suffer from major experiential deprivation in the social sphere. Thus, Altshuler (1971) refers to a "deficit in general experience," especially interpersonal.

To illustrate, let us take a closer look at the social situation of the children in this day school for the deaf who are now entering adolescence. Most of the students come from homes where they are the only nonhearing person. Only a small minority, mostly those with milder hearing deficits, have achieved a level of oral-verbal communication sufficient to carry on a spoken conversation of any length. Most of the students rely on manual communication for conversation, yet in the large majority of homes no parent—indeed, no member of the family—knows sign language. The implications of this regarding many aspects of the parent-child relationship are apparent; from the point of view of experience, most of these children have never engaged in complex verbal social interchanges with their parents or siblings.

In school, where the children are surrounded by peers who sign, another form of social deprivation is observed; namely, in the only setting in which the children have the opportunity for spontaneous social communication, the opportunities for such experience are inadvertently suppressed. The imposition of normal restrictions on student spontaneity adopted from conventional classrooms has a unique impact on the classroom of deaf children. Only while directly and continuously looking at the teacher can the deaf child "listen." Looking away, even slightly, takes the child out of contact. Thus, students cannot look at each other without ceasing to attend to the lesson.

Social deprivation is further exacerbated by the educational philosophy of many schools for the deaf, according to which the relative educational backwardness of the students in language skills is combatted by an intensified program of teaching through the constant drilling of elementary material (Mindel and McCay 1971; Vernon and Koh 1970). In Schlesinger's words (1977), "school settings . . . frequently place a premium on immobility, very young children are expected to sit still for long periods, in order to observe the teacher vigilantly." Craig and Collins (1970), in their landmark study, found the preponderance of classroom communication was teacher oriented in the form of questioning, informing, directing, demonstrating, and correcting, while only a minute portion of classroom time was devoted to the teacher listening to students in a nonjudgmental capacity or encouraging the expression of ideas by the students. Craig and Holman (1973) stated, "In schools for deaf children . . . creative and concrete student activity is frequently skipped over in order to get to the 'business of education.' "

My own observation is that the children, including the early adolescents, are moved from one structured classroom setting to another from the moment they arrive in school until the end of the day; they have little informal time, except for a brief lunch period. After school they board buses to return to an environment largely devoid of opportunities for social communication. Ironically, therefore, the only social setting in which these children would have a chance to develop social skills and ease in a group milieu suppresses opportunities for such experience. I found repeatedly that the resultant pent-up need on the children's part for "socializing" was a significant factor in most of the milder behavior problems in the classroom and between classes, particularly for the adolescents.

PSYCHODYNAMIC FACTORS: NARCISSISTIC VULNERABILITY AND DEFENSES AGAINST SHAME AND LOW SELF-ESTEEM

Deaf early adolescents are particularly prone to problems with self-esteem. At home there is often no one to listen to or appreciate their thoughts. Because of the absence of communicative reciprocity, they are often relegated to the periphery of family life and are denied a "voice" in family discussions. Frustration and narcissistic rage frequently result. Tantrums or deviant behavior may then be resorted to as attention-getting maneuvers; however, this inevitably leads to an increase in the parents' sense of futility about and impatience with their child. In addition, it has been found that hearing parents of deaf children tend to resort to shaming and autonomy-reducing coercion as means of setting up external controls (Schlesinger and Meadow 1972). For all those reasons, many deaf youngsters inherit, from their family situation, a devalued self-image, a propensity for shame, feelings of interpersonal futility, and proneness to narcissistic outbursts of rage.

The larger social milieu, of which the deaf adolescent is becoming increasingly aware, also presents an enormous challenge to self-esteem regulation. It is at this time that the reality and permanence of their defect strike home to these early teenagers with full and painful impact. The adolescent must confront, for the first time, the conflict over whether to reveal or conceal his deafness in public places. He may "pass" if he keeps his mouth shut and either pretends to understand or avoids situations likely to lead to exposure. Attempting to "pass," however, has pitfalls of its own, as the adolescent then risks misunderstanding situations and making embarrassing mistakes. Risking feelings of shame, either way, the solution chosen is often to "be cool": to act in control, to avoid interpersonal risks, and to conform superficially. Even deaf children of deaf parents, who have benefited since earliest childhood from a conflict-free avenue of communication and identification with their parents, and who have consistently been shown to have higher self-esteem than the deaf children of hearing parents, encounter narcissistic stress upon entering adolescence (Mindel and McCay 1971; Vernon and Koh 1970).

A related problem concerns children with a milder hearing deficit and substantial oral skills who, upon entering the preadolescent phase, begin distancing and "disassociating" themselves from the "deaf kids." These students reject peer interaction and attempt, usually maladaptively, to attract the attention of hearing teachers and to assert, by their behavior, "I'm not one of these deaf and dumb kids." Some of these students become overtly rebellious about attending a school for the deaf and develop problems with truancy or defiant attitudes in the classroom.

These grave problems with shame and low self-esteem may occasionally be observed directly; however, it is more common for aggressive and coercive behavior to be used as a defensive facade. The author's group-therapy experience provided numerous clinical examples of how defenses against narcissistic injury were manifested superficially as indifference to others, lack of empathy, and general callousness toward the feelings of peers.

CLINICAL EXAMPLE

Jim, a husky, well-developed boy who suffered from a superimposed language disability and who had, as a result, by far the poorest abilities in the group, was continually frustrated as a result of being ignored by his peers whenever he attempted to speak. This callousness seemed extreme, and repeated efforts were made by the therapist to call attention to it. Finally, one of the most capably communicating and popular boys said the unspeakable—namely, that Jim signed badly and that it was very hard to understand him. Previously, no one had been able to mention Jim's obvious problem. In the discussion that ensued, it became clear that the group members did not want Jim to talk and that his talking made them very impatient and irritated. In the subsequent group session, Jim was again ignored, but this time, instead of retreating into passive, smouldering silence, he said haltingly, but with great feeling, "I know I can't speak very well but why can't you try and understand me." Another boy replied that he just couldn't stand to watch Jim sign.

At this juncture, I pointed out that something puzzling was going on. The boys reacted to my clumsy efforts at signing with the utmost tolerance and interest; and yet, toward Jim, whose signing was far superior to mine, they showed intolerance. The boys rejoined that I was hearing and they liked the idea that I was trying to sign. Finally one brave youngster brought out the truth, namely, that Jim's signing looked "dumb" and he felt (the others concurred with great enthusiasm) that I would think they were all *dumb* and *retarded*. I commented that I knew perfectly well that none of them was retarded but that seeing Jim struggle must have reminded them of when they were little and could hardly speak. They must have worried at that time that people would think they were dumb. This interpretation had a significant impact on the group. Another boy in the group who was unusually talented, compared with the others, in his language skills—and who, in fact, surpassed the interpreting counselor in his ability to understand Jim's communication—appointed himself as translator and helper to Jim, something which Jim gratefully accepted. Both Jim and his "helper" were reported by the school staff at the end of the year to be improved in their social and behavioral adaptations.

Much has been written about the lack of empathy and concern for others manifested by deaf adolescents. In this author's experience, "lack of empathy" was often a "be cool" disguise serving as a defense against shame based on *overidentification* with the perceived defects of peers. By denying similarity of experience and feelings, they could disassociate themselves from painful feelings of depreciation and inadequacy. Sarlin and Altshuler (1968) found the thirteen- to fifteen-year-old deaf boys with whom they attempted group therapeutic work to be "preoccupied with violence and retaliation." In the light of present understanding of the psychopathology of self-esteem regulation, we can now see that these "preoccupations" represent narcissistic rage reactions to constant and painful reexperiencing of personal inadequacy, failure, and the inability to gain a receptive audience when expressing one's thoughts and feelings.

The school experience for all but the most academically successful deaf adolescents is one of continuous narcissistic stress. The thirteen- and fourteen-year-old boys I worked with were all keenly aware that they were reading below grade level, yet most of their academic day was taken up with drilling in elementary reading and language skills. Prevocational training or other hands-on activities such as crafts or shop, areas in which they were more likely to achieve some immediate success, were not emphasized in their program. Their awareness of their low skill level was all the more painful to them in the context of the heavy emphasis on their academic achievement.

In my opinion, the denial to these adolescents of experiences which could lead to feelings of accomplishment and mastery, combined with a constant emphasis on the areas of greatest weakness and deficiency, was a significant causal factor in their rebellious and aggressive behavior problems. Failure to provide experiences of competence and mastery in the school situation may also be a significant factor in the extremely high school dropout rate among deaf adolescents.

NEUROPSYCHIATRIC FACTORS: THE USE AND PROCESSING OF SIGN LANGUAGE IN A SOCIAL GROUP CONTEXT

It was evident from the conduct of the psychotherapy group, as well as from observations made in the classrooms and in more informal situations, that factors relating to the particular nature of signed communication played a significant role in group social interactions. In general, a decreased capacity to receive communication and to maintain attention to the communication of others seemed evident in group contexts. Part of this problem may be inherent in deafness and the consequent reliance on vision for "listening." While, for the deaf person, visual attention is being focused on one person's speech, others' communication coming from the peripheral visual field or from outside the visual field is lost. Myklebust (1964) has described the natural division of labor in the hearing person by which, while vision is focused on a particular object or event, audition takes over as a background scanning sense. The absence of such a scanning sense interferes with free-wheeling communicative interaction in group settings. The rate of signing, angle at which people are facing toward or away from each other, and lighting conditions all exert a powerful influence on the ease and flexibility of maintaining an informal group conversation (Caccamise, Hatfield, and Brewer 1978).

In addition to these inherent spatial and foreground/background problems, neuropsychologic factors further compromise group communication. Half of the boys in the group were deaf due to rubella. Vernon and Koh (1970) have reported that a high percentage of rubella-deaf youngsters have learning disabilities—one of the infrequent problems in language processing (receptive and/or expressive) which, when superimposed on the language deficit secondary to deafness, may go unrecognized. One boy in our therapy group had a major problem with this, and two others had a sizable deficit which interfered moderately with their communicative functioning.

There is increasing evidence that the CNS processing of sign language involves a more complex coordination of cerebral pathways than the processing of auditory language. For example, signed verbal information is first stored for the deaf in the visual iconic memory area which retains information for briefer duration than the short-term auditory system. This information must then be transferred to the auditory side for longer-term storage. These considerations have been reviewed recently by Caccamise et al. (1978), Kelly (1978), Stuckless (1978), and Wilson, Rapin, Wilson, and Denbury (1975). While these neuropsychologic processing factors may not interfere with the short conversational format, they may result in some tendency to fatigue or loss of efficiency in the reception of more lengthy discourse. An example of this was provided by Norwood (1978), who presented a videotaped news broadcast to a large group of deaf adults. A comparison was made between their viewing the broadcast with printed captions and their viewing the broadcast with simultaneous sign language interpretation. It was found that those who had viewed the captioned version had much better information recall than those who had viewed the signed (interpreted) version. Most of the subjects expressed a preference for captions, despite the fact that many of the subjects had a relatively low level of literacy.

Thus, complications arising from the spatial aspects of communication by sign language in groups, from the frequent occurrence of language-processing disorders, and from neuropsychologic limiting factors in the use of sign language—all combine to make signed communication in a group setting more arduous and difficult to sustain.

Summary

In this chapter I have reviewed observations from clinical consultation and group-therapy work with early adolescent deaf boys in a special day school for the deaf. I have stressed how problems in communication exert a profound effect on the lives of these youngsters, both by virtue of their past and present influence on family life and by their ongoing effect on peer-group processes and academic adjustment. Primary consideration was given to certain "here and now" aspects of these boys' lives: ongoing problems in the social fabric of their home and school; narcissistic vulnerabilities and defenses against shame; and language-processing difficulties. The ways in which these problems undermine the supportive effect of the peer group at a time when it plays a particularly important role in development were reviewed. By emphasizing current sources of difficulty, using a biopsychosocial approach, I hope to point out fruitful opportunities for significant psychiatric intervention in a psychiatrically vulnerable population whose needs for professional service have never been met.

REFERENCES

Altshuler, K. Z. 1971. Studies of the deaf: relevance to psychiatric theory. *American Journal of Psychiatry* 127:1521–1526.

Altshuler, K. Z. 1978. Toward a psychology of deafness. *Journal of Communication Disorders* 11:159–167.

Altshuler, K.; Deming, W.; Vollenweider, J.; Rainer, J.; and Tendler, R. 1976. Impulsivity and profound early deafness: a cross cultural inquiry. *American Annals of the Deaf* 121:331–345.

Caccamise, F.; Hatfield, N.; and Brewer, L. 1978. Manual/simultaneous communicative research: results and implications. *American Annals of the Deaf* 123:803–823.

Chess, S., and Fernandez, P. 1980. Do deaf children have a typical personality? *Journal of the American Academy of Child Psychiatry* 19:654–664.

Chess, S.; Korn, S.; and Fernandez, P. 1971. *Psychiatric Disorders of Children with Congenital Rubella.* New York: Brunner/Mazel.

Craig, H., and Holman, G. 1973. The "Open Classroom" in a school for the deaf. *American Annals of the Deaf* 118:675–685.

Craig, W. N., and Collins, J. L. 1970. Analysis of communicative interaction in classes for deaf children. *American Annals of the Deaf* 115:79–85.

Desmond, M.; Montgomery, J.; Melnick, J.; Cochran, G.; and Verniand, W. 1969. Congenital rubella encephalitis: effects on growth and development. *American Journal of Diseases of Children.* 118:30–31.

Desmond, M.; Wilson, G. S.; Melnick, J. L.; Singer, B.; Zion, T. E.; Rudolph, A. J.; Pineda, R. G.; Ziai, M. H.; and Blattner, R. J. 1967. Congenital rubella encephalitis. *Journal of Pediatrics* 71:311–331.

Edelstein, T. 1978. Development of a milieu interventive program for treatment of emotionally disturbed deaf children. In *Mental Health in Deafness.* Experimental Issues no. 2, Fall. National Institute of Mental Health, DHEW Publication no. (ADM) 79-524.

Freedman, D. A. 1980. Speech, language and the vocal-auditory connection. Paper presented at the Annual Margaret Mahler Symposium, Philadelphia, May.

Freeman, R.; Malkin, S.; and Hastings, J. 1975. Psychosocial problems of deaf children and their families: a comparative study. *American Annals of the Deaf* 120:391–405.

Fuhrer, L., and Litoff, S. 1979. Group intervention with hearing impaired adolescents in a high school setting. Paper presented at meeting on Mental Health Problems of Deaf Adolescents, Model Secondary School for the Deaf, Gallaudet College, Washington, D.C., June.

Furth, H. G. 1966. *Thinking without Language: Psychological Implications of Deafness.* New York: Free Press.

Galenson, E.; Miller, R.; Kaplan, E.; and Rothstein, A. 1979. Assessment of development in the deaf child. *Journal of the American Academy of Child Psychiatry* 18:128–142.

Goldberg, B.; Lobb, H.; and Kroll, H. 1975. Psychiatric problems of the deaf child. *Canadian Psychiatric Association Journal* 120:75–83.

Hicks, D. E. 1970. Comparison profiles of rubella and non-rubella deaf children. *American Annals of the Deaf* 115:86–92.

Jensema, C., and Trybus, R. 1975. *Reported Emotional/Behavioral Problems among Hearing Impaired Children in Special Educational Programs: United States, 1972–1973.* Series R, no. 1. Washington, D.C.: Gallaudet College, Office of Demographic Studies.

Kelly, R. 1978. Hemispheric specialization of deaf children: are there any implications for instruction? *American Annals of the Deaf* 123:637–645.

Lesser, S., and Easser, R. 1972. Personality differences in the perceptually handicapped. *Journal of the American Academy of Child Psychiatry* 11:458–466.

Levine, E. S. 1976. Psychological contribution. *Volta Review* 78:23–33.

Meadow, K. 1975. The development of deaf children. In E. M. Hetherington, ed. *Review of Child Development Research,* vol. 5. Chicago: University of Chicago Press.

Meadow, K., and Schlesinger, H. 1971. The prevalence of behavior problems in a population of deaf school children. *American Annals of the Deaf* 116:346–348.

Mindel, E. D., and McCay, V. 1971. *They Grow in Silence: The Deaf*

Child and His Family. Silver Spring, Md.: National Association of the Deaf.

Murphy, N., and Trybus, R. 1975. Hearing impaired school-learners. *American Annals of the Deaf* 120:86–91.

Myklebust, H. R. 1964. *The Psychology of Deafness*. 2d ed. New York: Grune & Stratton.

Naiman, D.; Schein, J.; and Stewart, L. 1973. New vistas for emotionally disturbed deaf children. *American Annals of the Deaf* 118:480–487.

Norwood, M. 1978. Comparison of an interpreted and a captioned newscast. Doctoral diss. University of Maryland. Cited in E. R. Stuckless. Technology and the visual processing of verbal information by deaf people. *American Annals of the Deaf* 123:630–636.

Rainer, J. D. 1969. Interpretation, communication, and understanding. In J. Rainer, K. Altshuler, F. Kallman, and W. Deming, eds. *Family and Mental Health Problems in a Deaf Population*. 2d ed. Springfield, Ill.: Thomas.

Rainer, J. D. 1976. Some observations on affect, induction, and ego development in the deaf. *International Review of Psychoanalysis* 3:121–128.

Rozek, F.; Sien, S.; Nostoff, P.; and Nower, B. 1979. The therapeutic classroom for deaf adolescents. Paper presented at the meeting on Mental Health of Deaf Adolescents, Model Secondary School for the Deaf, Gallaudet College, Washington, D.C., June.

Sarlin, M., and Altshuler, K. 1968. Group psychotherapy with deaf adolescents in a school setting. *International Journal of Group Psychotherapy* 18:337–344.

Schein, J. 1975. Deaf students with other disabilities. *American Annals of the Deaf* 120:92–99.

Schlesinger, H. 1977. Treatment of the deaf child in the school setting. In *Mental Health in Deafness*. Experimental Issues no. 1, Fall. National Institute of Mental Health, DHEW Publication no. (ADM) 77-524.

Schlesinger, H. S., and Meadow, K. P. 1972. *Sound and Sign: Childhood Deafness and Mental Health*. Berkeley and Los Angeles: University of California Press.

Siple, P.; Hatfield, N.; and Caccamise, F. 1978. The role of visual perceptual abilities in the acquisition and comprehension of sign language. *American Annals of the Deaf* 123:852–856.

Stern, D. N. 1978. The role of audition in the development of affect. Paper presented at Institute on Infant Psychiatry, American Academy of Child Psychiatry, New York, June.

Stuckless, E. R. 1978. Technology and the visual processing of verbal information by deaf people. *American Annals of the Deaf* 123:630–636.

Vernon, M. 1967. Characteristics associated with post-rubella deaf children. *Volta Review* 69:176–185.

Vernon, M., and Koh, S. 1970. Early manual communicative and deaf children's achievement. *American Annals of the Deaf* 115:527–536.

Williams, C. C. 1970. Some psychiatric observations on a group of maladjusted deaf children. *Journal of Child Psychology and Psychiatry* 11:1–18.

Wilson, J.; Rapin, I.; Wilson, B.; and Denbury, F. 1975. Neuro-psychologic function of children with severe hearing impairment. *Journal of Speech and Hearing Research* 18:634–652.

12 SPECIAL PROBLEMS IN BORDERLINE ADOLESCENTS FROM WEALTHY FAMILIES

MICHAEL H. STONE

The VIP status is often associated with special problems in therapy, since the VIP patient may expect the same privileges and bending of the rules from his therapist as those accorded him by the outside world. For our purposes, VIP connotes those whose wealth, position, fame, or talent renders them socially prominent or powerful. Younger patients rarely possess these qualities in their own right: the VIP adolescent is "special" only to the extent that his parents are special. Of the admittedly rare attributes that can confer VIP status, wealth will be encountered more often (at least in our culture) than the others. The ways in which wealth may affect psychiatric treatment deserve our attention, partly because many therapists will at some time have experience with patients from wealthy backgrounds, and because the attendant difficulties illustrate—in dramatic terms—problems relevant to less rarefied bands of the socioeconomic spectrum.

According to Brody (1969), the majority of Freud's patients came from economically privileged backgrounds. Some came from families of great wealth. The most notable example is that of the Wolf-Man (1918), who grew up on an estate in pre-Revolutionary Russia that measured approximately 210 square miles. Similar socioeconomic status was enjoyed by a number of the "as-if" patients described in Helene Deutsch's 1942 paper. There has probably always been an

Paper presented at American Society for Adolescent Psychiatry, May 16, 1977, meeting at Toronto.

overrepresentation of the affluent among the ranks of patients receiving analytic and analytically oriented psychotherapy, if for no other reason than the cost engendered by the frequent visits and the long time span. Not much attention was paid in the analytic literature, however, to the impact affluence might have on symptom formation or treatment, apart from isolated papers by Grinker (1977), Main (1957), Weintraub (1964), Wixen (1973), and myself (Stone 1972, 1979; Stone and Kestenbaum 1975). Some of the problems to which persons from extremely affluent families seem more than ordinarily vulnerable relate to parental deprivation and its aftereffects, to pathological narcissism, to impaired work motivation because of diminished need, and to certain forms of anti-social behavior that may go on unchecked because of a wealthy family's ability to smooth over run-ins with authority.

This chapter is concerned with possible adverse effects of extreme affluence on personality development in adolescents who appear to function at the borderline level. The criteria for defining this level are primarily those set forth by Kernberg (1967, 1977, 1981), although, as I have expressed elsewhere (Stone 1981), it is often difficult to establish with conviction a "borderline" diagnosis in this age range. Troubles in the sense of identity—the latter constituting the touchstone of border-line function—are so common in adolescents who seek psychiatric help as to render quite problematical the task of drawing a dividing line between neurotic-level adolescent turmoil and the pervasive and sharp contradictions in identity-sense that characterize borderline pathology. If we focus our attention, however, on the more extreme examples, where there can be no question about the severity of the identity dis-turbance, we can make a good case for the existence of "borderline" adolescents, many of whom go on to exhibit borderline function as young adults or to develop certain syndromes (anorexia nervosa, atypical but major affective disorders) that are usually within the bor-derline domain (Fard, Hudgens, and Welner 1978).

I maintain careful records of all the patients I have seen in office practice since 1966, from which I have been able to extract five border-line psychotherapy cases where the family had great affluence; three of these concerned adolescent patients. In addition, I saw in consultation or brief therapy two other adolescents from such families.

The following clinical vignettes will, I hope, highlight some of the problems that one is especially apt to encounter in treating borderline adolescents from backgrounds of extreme wealth.

Impediments in the Formation of Identity

A fifteen-year-old boy was referred for consultation because of a widening discrepancy between his scholastic achievement and his apparently superior intelligence. The problem was brought to the attention of his parents by the school authorities, who first noticed this "underachievement."

The boy showed considerable contempt for schoolwork, had no goals for the future other than "to see the world," and had begun to get into trouble at school, through a combination of "sloughing off" in his homework and aggressive behavior toward some of his schoolmates. This deterioration in his behavior had begun half a year before the consultation and had spread to include his parents, with whom he was also contemptuous and negativistic. He was particularly scornful of his parents' ambition that he become a physicist—a profession in which he had not the slightest interest—as requiring too much study and offering not enough pay. "Work sucks" was his succinct, if indelicate, commentary upon the parental frenzy over his indolence.

The son was aware of his father's "shady" business dealings that had led to immense wealth within the past several years, and this awareness contributed to his disdainful attitude. A year earlier, the father had set up a million-dollar trust for the patient, to be activated on his twenty-first birthday. This was no secret, since the father boasted of it continuously to anyone within earshot. As a result the boy could not help realizing that work and achievement were absolutely irrelevant for him, since, even if he did nothing, he would, in six years' time, be better off than almost everyone he knew. Yet he kept this realization under wraps, as it were, and seemed quite surprised when I pointed out how his father's flaunting of the trust fund had undermined his motivation to apply himself to anything and had effectively brought his personal development to an end. He had not even grasped how his flippant remarks about work were born of his parents' unwise decision which, in his case, had, with one stroke, removed purposefulness from his life and replaced it with futility.

Since the power of mere words is relatively limited in counteracting the effects of a large trust fund (what could I have said about the glories of work well done that might attract him away from the prospects of *la dolce vita?*), I urged the father to alter the trust so that his son could not enjoy the use of it until he reached thirty-five. Furthermore, necessity being the only antidote to wealth, I counseled the father to dole out only the most modest allowance in the intervening years. In this way, the patient could no longer have the "luxury" of frittering away his life. The parents accepted this advice—which, when they somewhat reluctantly put it into operation, had the salutary effect of propelling their son toward serious study and a useful career. Eight years later I was to learn that, although still arrogant and abrasive, he had achieved a good measure of psychological and financial independence—not as a physicist, but as an architect.

Problems in Limit Setting in the Face of Antisocial Tendencies

In an earlier paper (Stone 1972), I have commented on the ease with which wealthy families can bail out (literally) a child who has gotten into trouble with the law. Parents may find themselves, in their efforts to avoid scandal, trapped in a situation where each last-minute rescue only contributes further to the child's antisocial proclivities, demonstrating to him again and again that he can get away with anything. In cases of this kind, a night in jail may accomplish more than a year in therapy.

The following case concerns a nineteen-year-old borderline adolescent whose antisocial tendencies had already led to some difficulties with authority (he had been ousted from two schools because of drug abuse and petty thievery), but whose main problems were ennui and aimlessness. The more frantic his parents' efforts to impart some structure to his life, the more he rebelled, and the more chaotic his life became. The youngest of three children born to a highly successful manufacturer and his independently wealthy wife (whom he had divorced when the patient was nine), he lived sometimes with his brother and sister in a town house the parents had purchased for them (as a kind of trust) and sometimes in a cold-water flat he maintained out of his allowance. His parents had encouraged him to work; his father even entertained the hope his son would one day take over the factory. But the young man was insolent toward his employers, chronically late, and rude with the customers—with the predictable result that he never held one job more than a few weeks. The allowance was always forthcoming, and one or another parent could always be counted on for extra money. He still fancied himself as successor to his father's business, despite never having made any effort to learn its details.

I undertook to treat him, more at his parents' insistence than out of any genuine concern on his part, and noted that, although affable superficially, he was glib, unmotivated, and emotionally inaccessible. Grandiosity, entitlement, and other attributes of narcissistic character pathology were present to a marked degree. He kept only half his appointments. On the few occasions when I arranged meetings with him and his parents, he was extremely argumentative with them and they with each other. Each tried to manipulate the other two—and myself; no plan of action could be agreed upon. My explanations about how he played one off against the other, while pursuing his structure-less existence, met with polite nods of comprehension—but did *not* succeed in creating, in the parents, a "united front" impervious to his entreaties, much less instill in him any sense of goal directedness.

Psychological tests revealed a verbal IQ of 98 with a performance IQ of 105. It may be that the discrepancy between his modest endowment and the rather lofty aspirations the family had once maintained had contributed to his character pathology. He could never manage a large industrial concern—nor could he ever feel proud unless he did so. The idea of performing well at something much more humble was intoler-able to him. Therapy made no inroads into this unrealistic attitude. He far preferred doing nothing and preserving his illusions intact to doing something "menial" and having his illusions shattered.

I induced the parents to set up a "spendthrift trust"—which dis-pensed a sum every week to him sufficient for his needs. Along with this I got them to promise they would refuse all requests for extra funds, even if the alternative were jail or a flophouse. They were to encourage work of any kind but were to stop tantalizing him about taking over the family business. They readily agreed to these recom-mendations, though I have no idea how scrupulously they carried them out or what effect, if any, these measures might have had upon their son. After the session in which I announced this plan, the patient quit therapy, and I have never heard from any of them since.

Parental Deprivation and Its Aftereffects

A student of nineteen was referred for psychotherapy because of severe depression and suicidal threats that had begun to interfere with her college work. In addition, she had considerable uncertainty about her life goals. Confusion about sex identity was considerable, but this problem had less immediacy about it than the first mentioned. Her tendency to overspend and overeat when depressed was quite pronounced, as was her inability to concentrate on her assignments, during these increasingly frequent spells of moodiness and despondency.

She was the youngest of four children in a family of immense wealth. They were the grandchildren of the founder of one of the largest manufacturing concerns in the country. But far from being pampered, in the way youngest children often are, she was neglected by both parents to an unusual degree. Her father seemed capable of relating only to his sons and even so lived much of his life in voluntary confinement within the bedroom of his palatial main residence. The patient was never permitted inside and actually saw her father only on one or two occasions during the last three years of his life. He died when she was seventeen. Her chief ambition had been to do something which might win either his attention or his approval. She failed in both pursuits while he was alive; now that he was dead, life seemed to her bleak and meaningless. Her mother was a vain woman—very much caught up in "society"—who had always relegated the care of the children to the servants. She was away for long periods of time at one or another of the family's three other residences.

When the patient was in her early teens, her brothers often ganged up on her, taunting her about her appearance (she was somewhat overweight) and at times abusing her physically. The servants had no power over the boys, and the parents either were unavailable, or, if they happened to be at home, left strict instructions that they were not to be bothered. The patient often sought refuge by "camping out" in a cave at the edge of the estate. There she would take large quantities of comics and Coca-Cola with which to assuage her loneliness.

At college the loneliness became more intense; she now resorted periodically to gorging herself (alternating with vomiting, to keep her weight within bounds). Sometimes she would go on spending sprees, buying expensive jewelry and antiques—haphazardly and without any attempt to create a coherent collection of some kind. She had no hobbies or special interests, in any case, such as might have lent some sense of purposefulness to this activity.

Although reasonably attractive, she felt ugly and was afraid of men. In her relationships with others, she oscillated between sporadic heterosexual relationships, which gave her no pleasure, and homosexual ones, which, while pleasurable, frightened her because of their negative social implications. Caught in this dilemma, she became seriously depressed and suicidal.

Therapeutically, the depressive aspects of her condition were fairly amenable to intensive psychotherapy. This, despite her tendency to slip off unannounced to one of the family's four homes on a day when a session was scheduled. Sometimes I would get a call from her mother, who was considerably more responsible in these matters than her daughter, assuring me that the latter had arrived safely in Florida—or Maine—or Nevada—and would definitely be back in time for Monday's session. But once her acute symptoms had subsided, the tenuousness of her object relations came into clear focus, as did her lack of motivation to explore further any of the central dynamic issues. Rather than associate, for example, to her recurrent dreams of homosexual activity with older women by way of coming to grips with the underlying feelings of deprivation, she took a "flight into health," becoming engaged to a man she had known only a short time. She married within a few months and moved to a different city, quitting therapy in the process. A year later, I learned from the referring physician, who maintained contact with the mother, that the patient's marriage had broken up. One of the factors had been her impulsive and inconsiderate manner of spending money. She gave her husband inappropriately expensive gifts and large sums of money in such a way as to make him feel humiliated and useless. He also felt alienated by her bulimia and vomiting, which were much more difficult to conceal within the setting of married life.

Pathological Narcissism

An eighteen-year-old college student was admitted for long-term intensive psychotherapy on an inpatient unit because of inability to concentrate on her studies, a variety of "psychosomatic" symptoms including globus hystericus, and a manipulative suicide gesture.

She was the only child of a couple that had divorced when she was four. Both parents came from "old wealth"; the father, in particular, was the scion of a family whose name was a household word. He had never worked, dividing his time among various sporting activities and charitable organizations. The mother, with whom the patient had remained after the divorce, did some art work and also devoted time to charitable pursuits. She affected the "grande dame," was experienced by most people (including her daughter) as imperious and aloof, and, despite efforts to push the patient into certain social settings or artistic interests, did not really relate to her as an individual. The patient became an extension of the mother's personality; her job, as it were, was to fulfill the mother's unrealized dreams of artistic distinction. As it turned out, she did not develop abiding interests of her own—having spent much of her life trying to realize two unrealizable ambitions: to succeed where her mother had failed (neither woman had any appreciable artistic talent) and to effect a rapprochement with her father (who was and remained indifferent to her). In the process, the patient's personality took on many of the features of Deutsch's (1942) "as-if" cases. Her relationships were characterized by shallowness and inconstancy. She used others for her own ends. Certain persons—including her previous therapist and myself—would be singled out temporarily as rescuers or father surrogates to be idealized. But this attitude would soon give way to contemptuousness. She went through a period of sexual promiscuity, generally choosing men who were both considerably older and sadistic.

She had felt very rejected, more by her father, of course, than by her mother, and now seemed to be taking the offensive—in rejecting other people with queenly hauteur and peremptoriness. Interpretations to this effect made little impact upon her, however, for the truth of the matter was that she had been caught up in this mechanism for so long, and had for so long been a vain and self-centered person, she seemed now to lack any genuine interest in, let alone fascination with, other people.

While in the hospital she did make some gains, insofar as her expectations concerning her father—and also her artistic pretensions—were whittled down to more realistic proportions. She made her peace with the fact that her father would never welcome her or bestow any warm attention on her; she grew to accept the fact that her talents were not such as to conduce to the kind of fame and stardom she once felt entitled to.

Her growing resignation about these forlorn hopes was accompanied by sufficient improvement in her general condition to permit release from the hospital. Her relationships were now less chaotic and destructive than before, but just as shallow and fleeting. After a few months as an office patient, she quit therapy and moved to a fashionable community in the West, where, as I heard several years later, she had become self-supporting as a window dresser.

Discussion

The problems that were highlighted in the clinical vignettes, relating to identity formation, deprivation, limit setting, and narcissism, are by no means confined to the wealthy, nor are they peculiar to the borderline, as opposed to neurotic, level of function. Nor is there any evidence that extreme affluence predisposes to the development of a borderline condition. I think it would be nearer the truth to claim that, if one came from a family of considerable wealth and exhibited, for whatever reason, borderline function, some of the above-mentioned problems would be at the forefront, clinically; and their expression would be more intense and their resolution more complicated than might have been the case had wealth not been a factor.

Thus, limit setting, which often presents difficulties with normal adolescents, may be harder to achieve when a family has the power to manipulate the environment in situations where ordinary families and their children must conform *to* the environment. I have worked with two borderline adolescents in trouble with the law because of passing bad checks. The father of one kept bailing out his son—who remained sociopathic and marginal. The other was finally persuaded to let his son spend a night in jail and have his wages garnisheed. This young man eventually made good his debts and stayed out of trouble. I recall, when requested as a consultant at a private psychiatric hospital, a seventeen-year-old boy from a wealthy family who had been apprehended on several occasions for breaking and entering. He had stolen some articles and fenced them for drug money. There were no signs of a psychiatric disorder, apart from sociopathy, yet his parents inveigled the police to have him placed in a hospital, as though for some depressive disorder, rather than in a correctional facility. This is an extreme example, to be sure, but problems in appropriate limit setting occur in much more mundane situations among offspring of the wealthy—as, for example, in the area of budgeting money. Borderline adolescents are often irregular about keeping appointments. Those from well-to-do homes may be particularly cavalier about their psychotherapy sessions, since they realize that, from a strictly monetary viewpoint, having to pay for a skipped visit does not make much of a dent in their parents' resources. It is for this reason I recommended (Stone 1972), in order not to take advantage of the parents, terminating treatment whenever two sessions in a row were skipped for frivolous reasons.

The customary ways of regulating an adolescent patient's environment center around home and school. Generally, the adolescent will be in therapy in the same locale as his school, even if his family lives far away. School authorities are usually quite cooperative, especially if faced with an aggressive "acting-out" student, in setting up a behavioral program, under the guidance of the therapist, suitable for the correction of whatever asocial tendencies the school may have observed. Parents, of course, cannot have the detachment and objectivity of school authorities. Inclusion of the parents may be the keystone to the treatment process, yet, with wealthy parents, cooperation may be difficult to achieve. The father may, for example, be a busy industrialist, an important man in the community, the demands on whose time make it next to impossible to conduct any kind of family therapy or periodic sessions with the parents. The mother may be a society figure inaccessible for similar reasons. It will not always be easy for the therapist to distinguish between genuine reasons for unavailability and merely impressive-sounding excuses. Tact, diplomacy, respect, and firmness will all be required of the therapist if he is to create an environment in which the parents recognize the importance of their role in the treatment—and agree to participate. Separate sessions just with the parents will often be necessary; even if they are divorced, they must be helped to achieve unanimity of attitude on crucial issues (regarding limits, acceptable behavior, appropriate allowance, etc.) so that the patient cannot take advantage of their conflicting viewpoints. Some of the interventions a therapist may find useful in dealing with wealthy parents have been elaborated in a previous paper (Stone 1972).

Closely connected with limit setting is the subject of discipline—not in the sense of punishment but in the sense of self-regulation and perseverance with tasks. Family wealth may contribute to the faulty development of inner discipline in borderline adolescents, some of whom are raised with little expectation that they will perfect any skills or acquire any profession. Too much is given to them and done for them. If circumstances change, and work becomes a necessity, it may, after the patient's years of coasting along, become extremely difficult to acquire the self-discipline required for either schooling or work. Psychotherapy is jeopardized by a deficit of this ego strength, since regularity of appointments is important, as is the ability to persevere during the inevitable periods when therapy becomes dry or anxiety provoking.

Family wealth may magnify the identity disturbance in a borderline youngster or may delay the process by which some stable sense of self might have been acquired. There may be simply no pressure to become anything. This was true of the girl in the third vignette, although in that instance lack of parental pressure was accompanied by a global indifference concerning the fate of the children on every level, not just the vocational. If one has scarcely been the recipient of a parent's concern or interest, one tends to have little regard for oneself, even for one's own life. It is not surprising that two of her brothers threw their lives away—one dying at twenty-one from an overdose of heroin; the other, at twenty-three in a motorcycle accident.

The formation of a solid sense of identity is one task connected with the narcissistic path of development. Closely related to this, perhaps separable only for heuristic purposes, are the tasks of delineating one's goals and ambitions and of establishing a fairly accurate appraisal of one's worth. The latter comprises learning how one is esteemed in the eyes of others (integration of which creates a realistic self-esteem) and learning the extent and limitations of one's talents and capabilities. All the currently popular definitions of borderline mark out a domain where significant impairments in these tasks are common. Among those reared in great affluence, these impairments may become exaggerated or else permitted to go on uncorrected for longer periods in adolescence than would be tolerated in ordinary households. In the home with unusual wealth, the disparity between what a young person of average abilities can accomplish and what his role models have, or appear to have, accomplished may be considerably greater than what one might encounter in a middle-class home. This disparity may intensify discouragement and contribute to a pathological narcissism. Several clinical forms may be encountered—including an outward grandiosity with a hidden self-contempt, or a facade of self-denigration covering over a core, created through identification with the wealthy forebears, of superciliousness and inflated self-estimation.

Borderline adolescents are more apt to come from families where one or both parents are highly disturbed—perhaps functioning themselves at the borderline level (Masterson and Rinsley 1975). This seems no less true where wealthy families are concerned. The destructive powers of a highly disturbed "borderline" parent whose potential to interfere in the lives of others (including a borderline adolescent son or daughter) is magnified by wealth may be truly formidable. Several instances of parents' hiring private detectives to spy on their children (at a cost far outside the reach of those in average circumstances) were described previously (Stone 1972). I have also encountered situations where the "splitting" typical of borderline object relationships took the form of a wealthy borderline father caning his children for minor offenses—while wearing a facade of saintliness before neighbors and other persons in his extrafamilial environment. Ideally, family therapy would be instituted in order to confront the borderline parent with the full range of his behavior. Sometimes the wealthy parent will be quite cooperative with the therapist, as per their usual pattern of "good form" and graciousness in dealing with outsiders. The same father who was described (not without cause) by his borderline eighteen-year-old daughter as an "ogre" for having caned her and her brothers proved very reasonable in therapy—and rapidly gave up his abusiveness. Just as often, however, the wealthy parent will prove to be arrogant and resist any therapeutic interventions. The situation is not always salvageable—as when the (borderline) father of an anorectic seventeen-year-old, overly attached to this daughter and threatened by any drive on her part toward independence, refused to let her go abroad with other members of her ballet troupe and finally stopped paying for her treatment.

Borderline adolescents from wealthy environments will be particularly prone to depression if, in the place of parental affection, one finds the inordinate emphasis on good "form" (at the expense of candor and genuineness) typical of such homes (Stone 1979). Deutsch (1942) has drawn attention to this emotional aridity in describing the backgrounds of some of her "as-if" cases. The paradoxical deprivation amid plenty may at times go well beyond what a therapist can resolve through an interpretive technique alone; some form of supportive treatment will also be indicated. A therapist cannot become a surrogate parent for adolescents of this sort; nevertheless, a therapist's genuine interest in the patient's homework assignments, extracurricular activities, and so on, displayed with sincerity and in a measured degree, may prove enormously encouraging and helpful. In this connection I think of a seventeen-year-old referred to me for treatment by the principal of a private school to which the patient had been sent by his parents. His personality had become markedly abrasive. In between bouts of melancholy, he tended to be verbally, even physically, abusive toward his parents, siblings, and classmates. His parents, who had been quite inattentive to him throughout his upbringing, were wealthy Europeans who had arranged for him to complete his education in the United States, ostensibly because of the superior programs available in some of our preparatory schools but in reality to gain the comfort of having an ocean between him and them. Once here, he was either too depressed to concentrate on his homework or too belligerent to be tolerated by the school. He had little motivation for therapy, never remembered a dream, never alluded spontaneously to an emotion of any kind, and in other ways frustrated my efforts to maintain an exploratory atmosphere in the sessions. I began to go over his English compositions with him, gave him some pointers about his math, and listened to him sing operatic arias (he was a gifted singer and hoped to make a career in opera). Within several months, both his deportment and his grades had improved dramatically. The principal called to ask me what sort of magic I was performing. I had not the slightest idea. I certainly was not doing anything I had been trained to do. He got me to give him what he most needed—without his being conscious of what he was up to and without my being aware at the time of what I was being coaxed into providing. Alpert (1959) would have called it—out of embarrassment, perhaps, at the unscientific nature of the transaction—a "corrective emotional experience." It seems safe now to call it by its right name: parenting.

Summary

Borderline adolescents from wealthy families pose a number of special problems in psychotherapy. The family may use great affluence to cushion the lives of their children in such a way as to diminish motivation for work, avocational pursuits, or anything requiring self-discipline. This in turn may exacerbate problems in the formation of *identity,* already impaired in the borderline adolescent. Antisocial tendencies may go unchecked because of the wealthy family's unusual ability to get around the authorities whenever its children are apprehended for an offense. Appropriate limit setting, imposed in ordinary families partly out of economic necessity, may fail to be imposed where family wealth has nullified the necessity for it. Parental deprivation, encountered often among the very poor, may also be seen among the wealthy, some of whom insulate themselves against their children to a marked degree, via household servants to whom almost all parental functions may have been allocated. From such deprivation, various character deformations may develop, including pathological narcissism. Clinical vignettes, illustrating these points and containing some suggestions for therapy, have been included.

REFERENCES

Alpert, A. 1959. Reversibility of pathological fixations associated with maternal deprivation in infancy. *Psychoanalytic Study of the Child* 14:169–185.

Brody, B. 1969. Freud's case-load. In H. M. Ruitenbeck, ed. *Freud as We Knew Him*. Detroit: Wayne State University Press.

Deutsch, H. 1942. Some forms of emotional disturbance and their relationships to schizophrenia. *Psychoanalytic Quarterly* 11:301–321.

Fard, K.; Hudgens, R. W.; and Welner, A. 1978. Undiagnosed psychiatric illness in adolescents. *Archives of General Psychiatry* 35:279–282.

Freud, S. 1918. From the history of an infantile neurosis. *Standard Edition* 17:7–122. London: Hogarth, 1966.

Grinker, R. R., Jr. 1977. Children of the rich. Paper presented at the American Psychiatric Association, Toronto, May 2.

Kernberg, O. F. 1967. Borderline personality organization. *Journal of the American Psychoanalytic Association* 15:641–685.

Kernberg, O. F. 1977. The structural diagnosis of borderline personality organization. In P. Hartocollis, ed. *Borderline Personality Disorders*. New York: International Universities Press.

Kernberg, O. F. 1981. Structural interviewing. In M. H. Stone, ed. *Borderline Disorders*. Philadelphia: Saunders.

Main, T. F. 1957. The ailment. *British Journal of Medical Psychology* 30:129–145.

Masterson, J. F., and Rinsley, D. B. 1975. The borderline syndrome. *International Journal of Psycho-Analysis* 56:163–177.

Stone, M. H. 1972. Treating the wealthy and their children. *International Journal of Child Psychotherapy* 1:15–46.

Stone, M. H. 1979. Upbringing in the super-rich. In J. G. Howells, ed. *Modern Perspectives in Psychiatry*. New York: Brunner/Mazel.

Stone, M. H. 1981. Borderline syndromes: a consideration of subtypes and an overview, directions for research. In M. H. Stone, ed. *Borderline Disorders*. Philadelphia: Saunders.

Stone, M. H., and Kestenbaum, C. J. 1975. Maternal deprivation in the children of the wealthy. *History of Childhood Quarterly* 2:79–106.

Weintraub, W. 1964. The V.I.P. syndromes: a clinical study in hospital psychiatry. *Journal of Nervous and Mental Disease* 138:182–193.

Wixen, B. 1973. *Children of the Rich*. New York: Crown.

13 LEARNING DISABILITIES AND THE COLLEGE STUDENT: IDENTIFICATION AND DIAGNOSIS

JONATHAN COHEN

> A freshman student's presenting problem at a counseling service: "I came to the counseling service because I'm having trouble concentrating. I just don't understand what I'm reading. . . . It's all piling up, and I'm getting nervous about it all."

One of the major presenting problems for the clinician in a university counseling and mental health service is work-related difficulties. Procrastination, concentration difficulties, and writing blocks are just a few of the many symptoms that are common fare and reflect any number of underlying conflicts and difficulties. There is a tendency to assume that work and learning disorders are psychogenic in nature because this is so often the case, and the diagnosis of specific cognitive deficits, or what are often referred to as learning disabilities, is overlooked. By "work disorder" I mean an inability to exert effort and/or produce academically. A "learning disorder" refers to an inability to learn (e.g., total school failure or inability to learn a foreign language). Both of these terms are descriptive and do not specify etiology. Here the term "learning disability" will refer to a learning disorder in which neuropsychological factors are at play. It is the result of a specific cognitive deficit which, theoretically, reflects some kind of neuropsychological dysfunction.

For a small but nevertheless significant number of students—including those who are high achievers—specific cognitive deficits interfere with, and at times interrupt, college- and graduate-level learning and work. It has been estimated that 6 percent of the 1982 freshman class is learning disabled (Astin 1983). Historically, there has been an expectation that if students were high achievers and were accepted to college, particularly academically rigorous ones, they could not be learning disabled. Even if a student had a history of learning disabilities, it was assumed that it would not significantly affect college learning or work. It has been only in very recent years that clinicians, educators, and researchers (e.g., Bellak 1979; Clark 1981; Cruick-shank, Morse, and Johns 1980; Frauenheim 1978; Kline and Kline 1975; Rudel 1981; Rutter 1978; Weiss, Hechtman, and Pearlman 1978) have realized that specific cognitive deficits are often not outgrown. They do in fact affect the learning process in college and beyond, as well as psychological processes (e.g., self-representation, self-esteem, conscious and unconscious fears and expectations), in subtle and striking ways.

This chapter will describe the most common signs of learning disabilities in the university student. Although I will be discussing relatively high-achieving college students with whom I have had the most experience (at the Columbia College Counseling Service and privately), virtually all of my discussion is applicable to late adolescents and young adults in general. Procedures for identification, screening, and diagnosis of cognitive deficits in the college student that interfere with learning will be reviewed along with some of the clinical implications of the diagnostic process and the difficulties and implications of the role of clinician-diagnostician within the university system.

Exactly what is meant by learning disabilities remains vague; it is a diagnosis primarily made by exclusion and discrepancy (Rudel 1980). It is beyond the scope of this paper to address fully the important and complex question of the nature of learning disabilities. Most clinicians and researchers accept the notion that there are neuropsychologically based cognitive deficits which interfere with learning. In order to call such a deficit a learning disability it is essential to determine that the following factors are not causing the cognitive deficit(s): psychological conflict, mental retardation, inadequate educational opportunities, environmental disadvantage, sensory impairment, or neurological disease.

We do not fully understand the etiology of learning disabilities. Although there is strong evidence that learning disabilities reflect neurological dysfunction (e.g., Benton and Pearl [1978]; Ochroch

178

[1981] for a review), this remains a hypothesis. No two learning disabilities are alike. The fact that researchers and educators have often conceptualized a particular type of learning disability (i.e., dyslexia) as a unitary condition has led to seemingly contradictory findings. A discrepancy between intelligence and achievement is a necessary component of the learning disability diagnosis. Perhaps the most difficult as well as the most thought-provoking dilemma facing the professional and the profession is the definition and assessment of intelligence and achievement.

In children, and even more so with late adolescents and young adults, we are often not sure what the exact symptoms of learning disabilities are, what causes them, and how to remedy them. We do, however, have a set of guidelines that can aid us in the identification process and a set of symptoms that, not uncommonly, interfere with learning and work in the college student.

The Identification Process

Identification of learning disabilities in the university student is a two-stage endeavor: initial screening and comprehensive neuropsychological diagnostic testing. Optimally, both steps should be conducted by a clinician who is well versed in neuropsychology and psychodynamic and developmental psychology. It is particularly important that the clinician have a working understanding of how subtle, unconscious psychodynamic factors may interface with a learning disability—for this is almost always the case. For example, a student may perform extremely well in a progressive high school or a less demanding public school, both of which often allow him to excel in areas of strength and avoid areas of weakness. However, he may have difficulty in an academically rigorous college, where he cannot so easily avoid areas of weakness, for psychological and/or learning disability–related reasons. If a specific learning disability does in fact underlie the college-level learning disorder, it is extremely likely that psychological concerns and conflicts will also be present secondarily. These concerns and conflicts may mimic and mask a learning disability, and the clinician needs to be able to distinguish psychogenic and neuropsychological factors in the identification process. (The important and often subtle psychological effects of learning disabilities in the college student are beyond the scope of this chapter and will be taken up in a subsequent publication.)

The screening process consists of data gathering in the following four overlapping areas: the nature and history of the (work- or learning-related) presenting problem; an educational history; a medical history; and a review of the student's current level of social, psychological, and academic functioning. The first evidence of a learning disability in college students is usually found in their reports of academic difficulty. It is important to note that this is not always the case. For example, a student may initially come to the counseling service because he is depressed; only on careful and comprehensive examination will the clinician discover that a learning disability contributes to feelings of inadequacy, damage, and having "lost" part of himself. This may occur whether or not the student is cognizant of the learning disability. It is important to be as detailed as possible about what specific work and learning tasks are difficult for the student.

Clinical experience and recent research (Farnham-Diggory 1980) suggest that it is important to break down and analyze the specific part functions of the given learning task. A "part" function refers to a basic building block of learning. For example, to read (which is a complex or "whole" function) we need to utilize the following series of part functions: letter recognition, phonic associates, sound blending, perceptual discrimination, long- and short-term memory, and left-right orientation, to name just a few. Although an analysis of part functions is always useful with children, one of the major reasons learning disability identification is difficult with late adolescents and young adults is that they have usually learned to recognize and compensate for their (part-function) deficits. Although an eight-year-old child may reverse letters or words in a striking and relatively consistent manner, the adolescent or adult will typically have learned to be hypervigilant and use a number of tricks to compensate, so that at the age of eighteen he may only occasionally slip and have a reversal. No one sign is indicative of a learning disability, with the exception of dysgraphia, which will be discussed below. As is often the case in any diagnostic endeavor, it is only when we see a characteristic patterning, historically and currently, of signs and symptoms that diagnostic hypotheses should be stated with any confidence.

Educational history often provides important information for the clinician during the process of screening and diagnosis. It is common for learning disabled persons to have had early school failures, and the nature of these difficulties (i.e., "I just could never learn to spell no matter how hard I tried" vs. "I kept failing science, I got so nervous with all the blood and stuff") should generate hypotheses suggestive of learning disabilities with or without psychogenic factors. In addition to evaluating how the student did in basic subject areas such as reading, math, spelling, and writing, it is important to look at the history of other school-related functions such as sound blending (being able to blend the sounds, like "c," "a," "t" into "cat") and learning phonic associates, particularly when the student presents with a reading disorder. It is also important to assess the following lines of development, which may reveal the existence of maturational lags: maturation of language in general and reading in particular; the development of motor skills, motility, awkwardness, and hyperkinesis (inability to inhibit motor behavior); right-left confusion or lack of orientation in relation to body, time, or space; perceptual development in both auditory (e.g., being able to discriminate like and different sounds) and visual spheres (e.g., confusing "b" and "d"); and immediate memory, both visual and auditory. Because it is developmentally normal for a four-year-old to reverse letters but unusual and diagnostically significant for a nine-year-old to do so, an understanding of psychological development in general and normative cognitive development in particular is essential for the clinician.

There are some students who have repressed the actual experiences of failure and frustration but recall being labeled "lazy" or "dumb," by others and/or self, in spite of a history of high achievement. For example, one student, when asked about early school experiences, initially reported that "it was all okay, except that I was very lazy." When this hardworking, high-achieving college student talked with his mother about these early years, she reported that he had in fact shown letter reversals and difficulty mastering sequencing concepts ("before" and "after"). She initially assumed it was because of laziness and only later learned otherwise. Psychodynamic factors played an important role not only in his forgetting about his early learning disability–related failures but also in his motivation to learn and perform. It is useful to understand what academic areas a student has liked and disliked over time, as this often reflects a pattern of strengths and weaknesses that may have diagnostic significance.

It is always important to examine a sample of the student's handwriting, especially writing from class notes (in which a student typically is not trying to "write nicely" for anyone) and on unlined paper.

Writing samples may reflect characteristic errors in spelling, punctuation, and grammar; sloppiness; and expressive difficulties that can be of diagnostic significance.

Medical history may also provide important diagnostic hypotheses. Head injuries, encephalitis, epilepsy, hyperactivity, and, to a lesser extent, lead intoxication and perinatal hazards have been correlated with learning disabilities (Heinicke 1971). Of course, gathering a medical history also allows one to rule out congenital or "acquired" visual or auditory acuity difficulties, which is necessary for a learning disability diagnosis to be made.

A review of the student's current level of social, psychological, and academic functioning is important for a variety of reasons. It provides an opportunity to assess to what extent psychosocial factors may be contributing to a learning or work disorder, which is so often the case. It also allows the clinician to begin to assess the student's achievement and ability. Although assessing achievement and ability is a complex task, one that is often difficult without comprehensive neuropsychological testing (even then it is sometimes problematic), in some cases a student will clearly have the required intelligence and motivation but experience significant difficulty with freshman English or mathematics or may demonstrate a striking discrepancy between abilities. For example, a student may score extremely high on the quantitative SATs but be unable to remember phone numbers. The SAT scores may also be a clue to ability-achievement discrepancy in several other ways. It is my impression that, for liberal arts students, an SAT quantitative-verbal score difference of greater than 150 points is diagnostically suggestive of a learning disorder. This may be indicative of a learning disability or psychogenic, economic, or cultural factors, or any combination of these. Receiving low or even average SAT scores (in the 400s) while performing at a very high level may reflect not only high motivation and sustained effort but also a learning disorder (Slack and Porter 1980).

Common Signs of Learning Disabilities

There are a variety of ways that academic functioning can be affected by specific cognitive deficits or learning disabilities. The college student with a learning disability is most commonly affected in language-related processes (reading, learning a new language, writing) and mathematics-related processes.

JONATHAN COHEN

LANGUAGE DISABILITIES

READING

Some students have had difficulty learning to read in childhood because of one of a number of specific cognitive deficits. A deficit in any one of the following basic building blocks or part functions can interfere with learning to read and the reading process: letter recognition, phonic associates, sound blending, perceptual discrimination, short- and long-term memory, left-right orientation, attentional shifting, and transmodal association. Bright children often learn to compensate for these difficulties with or without remediation. However, they will often *read slowly* and *not for pleasure* throughout their educational career and beyond. These are two of the important indications of a reading disability in the college student. Being a slow reader can become a significant constraint for the student who had performed well in a "relaxed," "easy," or "progressive" high school but is now in a high-powered and academically rigorous college where there is more work and less time to complete assignments.

The experience of being a slow reader can contribute to a sense of being dumb and inadequate. This psychological reaction to the deficit is a common one for many learning disabled students and often negatively affects academic as well as social expectations and experiences. In fact, for those students who have successfully compensated for their learning disabilities, these psychological concerns characteristically still plague them in spite of high achievement.

For example, with an eighteen-year-old student who was moderately depressed and having difficulty concentrating on his college work, it was unclear whether learning disabilities, as well as psychological concerns, were interfering with his ability to work. He reported that he had significant difficulty learning to read and reversed letters and numbers in childhood but that this now occurred only very rarely. Comprehensive testing revealed that he had a visual-spatial relations deficit which resulted in his occasionally reversing percepts (e.g., letters and words) and reading quite slowly. He was very bright and had a number of outstanding cognitive strengths. There was no indication that his cognitive (visual-spatial) deficit currently interfered with learning or work. In fact, his cognitive ability to learn was excellent. Diagnostic testing revealed that he had a well-integrated, inhibited obsessive-compulsive character with depressive tendencies and that his sense of self vacillated from that of a creative, likable, and gifted person to that of an inadequate, "damaged-in-the-head" boy whose products were "not good enough." When he thought about this, he became moderately depressed and felt he had "lost something." It became apparent that these feelings had contributed significantly to his plagiarizing in adolescence and his feelings that his own productions were not good enough. Plagiarizing resulted in severe storms of guilt and fearful anticipation of future writing assignments. These depressive concerns and anxious devaluing of his production (involved in his learning disability–related experiences) were exacerbated by developmentally normative freshman year separation-related concerns (Medalie 1981) and contributed to his current depression and concentration difficulties.

Reading comprehension is another learning disorder which may be the result of a learning disability. This is often particularly difficult to assess in the screening interview, and even at times with comprehensive diagnostic testing, because students have typically learned to compensate for the specific cognitive deficit to a large, but incomplete, extent. As a result, the behavioral manifestations (letter reversals) of the cognitive deficit (a left-right orientation deficit), which are often relatively easy to identify in childhood, are absent or quite difficult to discern in the college student. The following types of questions can help suggest factors related to learning disabilities and psychosocial problems that may interfere with reading comprehension: Has reading comprehension consistently been problematic? When did it begin? Is comprehension difficult with affectively laden reading content and/or neutral content? What seems to make it difficult (e.g., poor memory or word reversals or unempathic teachers), and what, if anything, has made it less of a problem? What other academic difficulties exist, and, if there are some, what does the pattern of difficulties suggest? Reading comprehension difficulties that reflect a learning disability typically have existed throughout schooling and are evident with all types of reading material. Depending on what specific deficits seem to lead to the comprehension disability (e.g., very poor immediate visual memory), one should be able to make predictions that are consistent with the deficit, for example, that the student would also have had difficulty remembering what was written on the blackboard.

LEARNING A NEW LANGUAGE

Most people—particularly bright ones—who experienced a reading disability in childhood usually learn to compensate for their deficit and become fluent, albeit slow, readers. It is not uncommon, however, for the learning disability to interfere significantly with the acquisition of other languages, be it a foreign language or a "new" language like the computer language FORTRAN. Many science classes involve learning a host of Latin and Greek terms and as such are also akin to learning a new language. Although a learning disabled student may compensate for a deficit, it seems that it does not "go away" but in fact may interfere with certain forms of new learning (Dinklage 1971; Rudel 1981). New-language learning appears to be one of the major examples of this, and it is a difficulty that may significantly affect the student's academic career. In fact, there have been students who have failed to receive their college degrees because they could not meet an undergraduate language requirement. It has also been suggested that a small, but significant, number of college dropouts can be attributed to this language problem (Dinklage 1971).

Various types of cognitive deficits can result in the college student's being unable to learn a new language. Certain deficits interfere with the student's being able to learn a foreign language with the audio-lingual method, and other deficits interfere with the more traditional methods that focus on reading and writing as well as listening and speaking. Among the many learning disabilities that can result in an inability to learn a foreign language are visual processing disabilities and auditory-related disabilities (see Dinklage [1971] for a more complete review and discussion of this issue). There are various types of visual processing deficits, of which strephosymbolia is a common one. A strephosymbolic disorder is characterized by a reversal of whole words (e.g., "saw" becomes "was") and does not always occur in a consistent manner. Children with this type of visual processing disability will commonly learn to compensate by being hypervigilant when they read, and they recognize when a particular word does not fit in the context of the sentence (e.g., "He *saw* sad"). However, the college-age student learning a new language has no means to discern whether a word "looks right" or fits, and as a result learning is inhibited. Given that listening is usually a central aspect of learning a new language, any kind of auditory disability, be it poor immediate memory or poor auditory discrimination, will seriously interfere with the process.

Psychological problems can also interfere with learning a new language, and some may initially mimic a learning disability. For example, one student reported that he had failed French twice and was now taking it for the third time because he felt he should learn to speak a foreign language. He was an extremely bright and verbal young man who complained of "comprehension" difficulties with regard to the written and spoken word and "mixing up my letters." However, during the screening process it became clear that he had no history of reversing letters or any associated signs (he had no difficulty in early schooling) but that he felt volcanic-like rage toward his father, who was a Romance language professor. For this young man, learning French involved a paternal identification and evoked powerfully conflicted affects and fantasies which interfered with his ability to learn French.

WRITING

There are two major forms of writing or dysgraphic difficulties that college students may show. Sloppy handwriting is often due to spatial relations difficulties and is not a language disorder per se. Since these difficulties rarely interfere with learning or work in college, they almost never come to the attention of the college counselor. The typewriter cures!

The second form of dysgraphia is more seriously disabling and difficult to remedy. In general, dysgraphia is characterized by marked spelling, grammatical, and capitalization errors as well as an inability to put one's thoughts on paper in an articulate manner, as opposed to verbal expression. This form of dysgraphia is a language disability that manifests itself in written communication and as such is sometimes referred to as reflecting a left-hemisphere dysfunction. College students with this form of dysgraphia may also have dyslexic difficulties. This can be somewhat confusing for teachers and college counselors who assume, incorrectly, that, if a student has difficulty writing, he will have difficulty reading.

A number of factors tend to characterize left-hemisphere dysgraphia. Spelling is typically horrendous, and, in a related fashion, spelling achievement level (as measured on the Wide Range Achievement Test) will be significantly lower than verbal IQ. The student's history will reveal difficulties with all written assignments (book reports and in-class essays), and a general avoidance of writing will usually be evident. One subtype of dysgraphia is characterized by phonetic spelling errors (dyseidetic type); the other major subtype is characterized by spelling errors that are not phonetic and writing that is, in fact, often difficult to decipher (dysphonic type). Many people have a combination of the two (mixed type).

In both subtypes of dysgraphia, spelling is poor overall. Simple words are misspelled ("he" for "her"), letters are often reversed ("b" for "d" and "clam" for "calm"), and homonyms are mixed up ("their" for "there"). Letters are juxtaposed ("wacth" for "watch"), similar-sounding vowels are confused ("a" for "o"), as are similar-sounding consonants ("d" for "b," "assemble"). Syllables may be omitted ("obvus" for "obvious") or added ("symiphony" for "symphony"). Capitalization and punctuation are usually poor and, at times, bizarre looking; for example, capital letters will be placed in the middle of a word. Handwriting is also often poor. Students may run words together, go off the line, and not use a consistent slant, as well as use a combination of cursive and print writing.

Although many students may have one or two of these difficulties, it is extremely rare to see a clustering of these signs in a nondysgraphic student with the random nature of errors that characterize dysgraphia. In other words, many students may use cursive writing and printing or make certain spelling errors, but in a consistent fashion, while the dysgraphic student makes these errors at random. Although college educators are bemoaning the nationwide lack of writing skills, a dysgraphic student is not simply lacking in certain writing-related skills or expressive ability. (In fact, many dysgraphic students develop loquaciousness and articulate verbal abilities to compensate for their deficit.) Further training and remediation often seem to be of little avail for the dysgraphic student. In fact, they may only exacerbate the frustration and sense of inadequacy that colors the self-image and self-esteem of so many learning disabled students.

An example is the student who came to the counseling service on the recommendation of his history professor, who had been perplexed at the marked discrepancy between his "extremely intelligent and articulate class comments" and a recently completed in-class essay which was described as "elementary school–level spelling errors, terrible punctuation, and a lack of articulateness." The student described having always had these kinds of difficulties. He had been tested at ages six and a half and eleven and was told on both occasions that psychogenic factors alone contributed to his writing difficulties. He had been in psychotherapy for several years, and his writing difficulties remained. A writing sample and his history of making certain characteristic spelling and grammatical errors suggested that he had a dysgraphic disability. He reported that he had always asked his mother or friends to edit and often type his papers. Because this student also showed moderately serious characterological conflicts, he was referred for comprehensive neuropsychological diagnostic testing to clarify and to begin to determine what neuropsychological and/or psychological factors were affecting his writing. The testing revealed that he was an exceptionally bright young man who was dysgraphic (dyseideitc type). In other words, he had a learning disability that interfered with his ability to write clearly, spell, and use grammar correctly, although he was quite able to articulate his thoughts orally. He also had psychological concerns, some secondary to the learning disability (i.e., he felt stupid, damaged, and inadequate) and some unrelated to the learning process and his disability.

A dysgraphic disorder affects learning in a variety of ways. The process of learning to write, to describe one's thoughts in a clear, orderly, and articulate fashion on paper, imposes a discipline on our cognitive processes that contributes to learning and growth in a very fundamental and general way. For the dysgraphic, this process represents a limited, not to mention terribly frustrating and upsetting, avenue of learning. There are other, more specific, and potentially critical implications of dysgraphia for the college student: note taking in class is often slow and burdensome, and in-class essays are extremely problematic, as is the essay requirement on major examinations like the LSATs.

MATHEMATICS DISABILITY

There are many cognitive disabilities which may contribute to difficulties in mathematics that are often referred to functionally as dyscalculia. The two most common factors that contribute to dyscalculia in the college student are deficits in short-term memory (auditory or visual) and visual-spatial orientation. Short-term memory difficulties are most often seen in subjects where "arbitrary" rather than "conceptual" memory is required, like mathematics, chemistry, and certain aspects of biology and physics. Short-term memory difficulties may be related to what Rudel (1980) describes as "a deficient capacity to actively encode incoming information according to useful classificatory schema." Some students who have a visual-spatial difficulty will report becoming confused in mathematics classes. A visual-spatial orientation deficit may reflect confusion about what is left versus right (and perhaps "before" and "after"), or a tendency to reverse or rotate visual percepts, for example, so that a diamond may look like a square. However, most college students who have a history of visual-spatial orientation difficulties do not report problems in mathematics because they have learned to compensate for these difficulties or to avoid math classes.

Dyscalculic students are seen less often in the liberal arts college counseling service than dyslexic or dysgraphic students because it is easier to avoid mathematics than reading or writing. Dyscalculic students may be seen somewhat more often at engineering colleges. Currently an engineering degree virtually insures a student a job after graduation and as such is a powerful lure for many. There are some students whose dyscalculic disabilities did not seriously interfere with high school work because it was relatively undemanding or easy to avoid difficult academic tasks. Engineering school, however, is typically highly demanding and rigorous, so a disability that affects mathematics quickly becomes a major issue.

Comprehensive Diagnostic Testing

Comprehensive neuropsychological diagnostic testing provides an opportunity to confirm the presence of a learning disability and describe the often complex and clinically important interaction between psychological and neuropsychological factors. Comprehensive testing is time-consuming and may be relatively costly; thus it is indicated only when necessary. For instance, if a student describes an educational history suggestive of a reading disability and currently reads slowly and not for pleasure but is functioning well in school and socially, diagnostic confirmation of a specific cognitive deficit that hypothetically underlies the slow reading will add little. Although it is beyond the scope of this chapter to examine psychotherapeutic and other treatment implications, it is important to note that it is often useful to communicate to the student that he may have a learning disability which has affected him educationally and, perhaps more important, psychologically. A therapeutic exploration of these issues (e.g., how the student has coped with this cognitive weakness; how it has affected his self-representation, expectations, and concerns) is often useful. If, however, it is difficult to distinguish psychological dynamics from possible neuropsychological factors, comprehensive testing may be warranted.

In addition, if confirmation of the presence or absence of a learning disability will significantly affect the student's career, comprehensive diagnostic testing is essential.

There is almost as much confusion about what constitutes an adequate neuropsychological diagnostic test evaluation as there is about the notion of a learning disability (Rothstein 1982). A comprehensive neuropsychological diagnostic process involves an examination and analysis of the following three areas: (1) intellectual and achievement levels, (2) neuropsychological factors, and (3) personality factors. It is naturally important to integrate this formal diagnostic process with history taking and a clinical interview. In the absence of this type of comprehensive assessment, a partial evaluation tends to determine the results, and important findings may be overlooked.

An examination of intellectual and achievement levels often begins with the administration of a standard IQ test (e.g., the Wechsler Adult Intelligence Scales [WAIS]) and achievement test (the Wide Range or California Achievement Tests). Although it is unclear whether IQ tests measure intelligence, it is well known that performance on these tests (e.g., WAIS) correlates highly with school performance. From a clinical point of view, an analysis of the student's strengths and weaknesses on the various subtests that make up an intelligence test is much more important than the IQ scores per se. Intertest and intratest analyses will often suggest which cognitive functions are relatively weak (e.g., immediate auditory memory) and why this may be so (perhaps anxiety or an auditory processing deficit that results in the student's scrambling what is heard). From further testing as well as talking with the student about test-taking experiences, one may discern a pattern of findings, which then provides a foundation for an overall diagnostic impression.

Grade level is difficult to assess in college and becomes a somewhat artificial measure. In addition, many achievement tests do not have norms that extend beyond the twelfth grade. Nevertheless, college students with learning disabilities typically function significantly below twelfth-grade level, and an analysis of mistakes made on achievement tests provides important data and hypotheses about what has contributed to a learning disorder.

An examination of neuropsychological functions should involve an assessment of the various cognitive part functions or basic building blocks of learning. The neuropsychological examination of part functions involves, among other things, an assessment of "soft" neurological signs. Most soft signs concern immaturities in developmental functioning, such as language, motor coordination, or perception. A patterning of soft signs is often used as evidence or an indication of brain dysfunction. Such signs are regarded as "soft" not because they are unreliable but, rather, because their interpretation and meaning remain somewhat uncertain. However, a series or patterning of soft-sign findings, in conjunction with other test findings, supports the diagnosis of a learning disability.

A variety of neuropsychological functions should be examined. Auditory discrimination abilities, visual processing mistakes ("b" for "d") and abilities (i.e., as measured by the Raven's Progressive Matrices), and tactile processing (graphesthesia and finger agnosia) are important sensory processing, neuropsychological functions that may underlie a learning disability. Immediate visual memory, as assessed by the Benton Test of Visual Retention or the Illinois Test of Psycholinguistic Abilities (ITPA) visual memory subtest, and immediate auditory memory, as assessed by the ITPA auditory memory subtest or the WAIS digit span subtest, are also important part functions that underlie many aspects of learning. Receptive and expressive languages are also basic neuropsychologically related processes.

An examination of personality functioning, with the Rorschach and TAT in conjunction with tests like the WAIS, provides an opportunity to understand not only the nature of the student's concerns, level of functioning, and self/object representation and conflicts but also the interrelationships between specific cognitive deficits and personality functioning. Although certain psychological concerns (e.g., feeling "dumb") may have developed originally from unconscious determinants as well as responses to specific cognitive deficits, it is often difficult to discern which factors inhibit learning in the here and now. In fact, usually a complex combination of the two is involved. In addition, psychological factors may appear to mimic or camouflage a learning disability. An analysis of personality function in conjunction with an educational, cognitive, and neuropsychological evaluation provides the only way to differentiate these factors. Even with this type of comprehensive neuropsychological diagnostic battery, diagnosis is by no means a simple endeavor.

Additional tests and diagnostic exploration may and should be added, as needed, to these basic ingredients of the neuropsychological testing procedure. For instance, if a student has difficulty reading, there are a variety of tests that measure very specific aspects of the reading process which may further clarify the nature of the disorder. Test scores on any one test are not good indicators of a learning disability (Coles 1978): a patterning of findings across tests and in a qualitative as well as quantitative manner provides a basis for valid diagnostic impressions.

DIAGNOSTIC IMPLICATIONS

The diagnosis of a learning disability for the college student is often therapeutic in and of itself. Understanding why learning and schoolwork have been difficult, be it in subtle or striking ways, and realizing that it is not because one is "dumb" are usually experienced as a relief. However, this diagnosis may also contribute to a sense of being damaged, helpless, and depressed. Moderate to severe depressive reactions are most often seen in students with long-standing, characterologically narcissistic concerns. It is not uncommon for students to experience simultaneously a sense of relief and of loss. Coming to terms with one's limitations as well as one's strengths is a central part of the identity formation process in the college years. It is always initially painful to accept weaknesses or limitations, particularly when they are related to highly valued processes. For most university students, intellectual functioning is, and has been, prized, and future occupational hopes rest on intellectual achievements. Recognition and acceptance of a cognitive deficit often result in the depressive experience of losing a valued part of oneself.

The diagnosis may also provide students with the opportunity to request a waiver for certain academic requirements, such as foreign languages or writing in-class essays. The fact that a learning disability diagnosis can be used to alter academic requirements and admissions procedures raises complex educational and philosophical questions. Section 504 of the 1973 Rehabilitation Act (Public Law 93-112) prohibits discrimination on the basis of handicap against persons in programs receiving or benefiting from federal funding. This law mandates equal opportunity for disabled college students, among others. It has been suggested that some modification of academic requirements and testing methods, as well as specific learning aids, will be needed if colleges are to comply with the law (Miller, McKinley, and Ryan 1979). However, if a university decides that its definition of a well-educated person involves, for example, knowing a foreign language, what right does the state have to alter this?

192

Clearly there are important social consequences to being diagnosed as learning disabled. Diagnosis is a labeling process with social implications, some detrimental and some beneficial, for the student. Most of the research in this area has been conducted with learning disabled children, where Rist and Harrell (1982) report that the label may lead to less positive classroom interaction with teachers, more teacher criticism, reduced levels of interaction with parents, more peer rejection, and a type of "learned-helplessness" syndrome. They report that the label may also provide benefits, such as special support and attention from teachers and parents. It is unclear what types of social implications this label may have for the college student.

Diagnosis also has important implications for remediation, which is complex for college students with learning disabilities. There are many different schools of thought about remediation and no consensus about which disabilities are remediable and which are not. In general, successful remediation programs help the student recognize and compensate for the disability. As learning disabilities are being increasingly recognized as a problem that plagues not only young children but late adolescents and young adults as well, there has been an increased effort to develop appropriate remediation procedures. For example, the National Institute of Education has funded a Learning Disabilities Research Institute at the University of Kansas with a focus on adolescents and young adults (Clark 1981; Schumaker, Deshler, Denton, Alley, Clark, and Warner 1981; Schumaker, Deshler, Nolan, Clark, Alley, and Warner 1981). Remediation and educational specialists are also reporting success in their work with late adolescents and young adults (e.g., Alley and Deshler 1979; Cruickshank et al. 1980; Miller et al. 1979; Siegel 1975). For disabilities such as dysgraphia, remediation is often of no avail, and the management is usually compensation. In other words, there usually does not seem to be any way to teach these language disabled students to express their thoughts on paper in a clear and articulate manner. Instead, it appears that they will need to continue to rely on scribes and dictating machines as compensatory aids. Because many colleges currently have no learning disability experts or programs, it is important that clinicians know that a growing number of colleges have developed special learning disability remediation programs (Gary 1981). Some colleges are specifically geared to the needs of moderately to severely learning disabled students (Fielding 1981).

Diagnosis may also suggest that short- or long-term psychotherapy be instituted. The student's cumulative reaction to the specific cognitive deficits, of which he may or may not have been conscious, often creates psychological concerns and inhibitions for which short-term therapy may be quite helpful. The learning disability experience may also have become an organizing experience for additional psychological difficulties (Pine 1980). For instance, a child's visual perceptual disability may contribute to early experiences of vagueness and confusion about the world. If the early experiences were managed by impulsivity, adaptation to later psychological conflicts may utilize these same psychological pathways. Although this is difficult to discern in a short-term therapeutic relationship, it may be useful to bear in mind when beginning to conceptualize the student's psychological development. Certainly in the course of psychoanalytic psychotherapy it may be helpful in direct reconstructive work with the student.

The Role of the LD Diagnostician in the University

The learning disability diagnostician in the college setting typically works within the college counseling service or mental health service. As such, the counseling service clinician's role in the screening and identification process reflects the role of the counseling service in the larger organizational system—the university. It is quite important for the counseling service staff not to confuse therapeutic and diagnostic roles, because the role of diagnostician may involve communication with deans and committees about the student. Confidentiality of the student-therapist relationship is fundamental to psychotherapy and counseling and essential for the development of a trusting and collaborative relationship. The diagnosis of a learning disability presents the counseling service with a dilemma, because communication of these findings to anyone may be for "the good of the student" but shatters confidentiality. If the service decides that this information is needed (e.g., by the dean) to make an administrative decision and the student gives permission for this to occur, the counseling service runs the risk of developing a reputation in the student body as a place to "get out of academic trouble."

If a student may have a learning disability and confirmation of this will be needed, perhaps for a waiver of an academic requirement, it is recommended that the student be seen for an "administrative evaluation." In other words, the student is told at the beginning that confidentiality will not be in effect and that if he wants diagnostic findings communicated to a dean or appropriate committee, this may be done.

Although this procedure may appear cumbersome or artificial, it maintains boundaries, protects the integrity and reputation of the counseling service, and, by extension, protects the students in the long run.

College deans often call on the counseling service for advice and support in a variety of situations. In fact, one of the functions of the college counseling service is to provide such support and consultation to the college's administrative staff. Since the study and management of learning disabilities among college students is a relatively new area, administrators will naturally tend to request and act on the clinician's findings and recommendations. There is a huge difference between reporting diagnostic findings and describing the consequences they will have in college learning and work, on the one hand, and making specific academic policy–related recommendations, on the other hand. Although it may be tempting and even requested, dictating academic policy is not the role of the university mental health professional. However, the mental health professional's role is complex because at times it is appropriate to make recommendations and, as a result, influence academic policy. The role of clinician in the university involves managing boundaries and clients different from those of the private practitioner. It is important to clarify whether the student or the administration is the "client" and to determine the nature of the task at hand.

Summary

The identification and diagnosis of a learning disability in the college student are complex tasks. They constitute important tasks when we realize that 720,000 college students (6 percent, if we assume that there are 12 million in college today) may be learning disabled (Astin 1983). It is evident that children with learning disabilities are at risk for psychological and social problems in adolescence and young adulthood (Bellak 1979; Crabtree 1981; Cruikshank et al. 1980; Horowitz 1981). There is a risk that the learning disability will not be identified, and, hence, the problem will be treated as only a psychogenic one. Unfortunately, this will tend to contribute not only to the student's feelings of guilt, stupidity, and inability to change but also to the clinician's sense of frustration.

The description of the learning disabled college student and the two-step identification process in this chapter provides guidelines to aid understanding of these issues. Most colleges have not yet come to grips with what it means to have learning disabled students in terms of teaching, academic evaluation, diagnosis, and college counseling. To do so is important not only because of recent laws that guarantee equal educational opportunity for these students but also because a learning disability, whether overt or covert, can profoundly affect a person's educational and psychosocial development. It has often been said that the capacity to love and work is the foundation for the healthy adult. It is easy to see how academic learning is the work of the college student and educational success or failure is linked integrally to self-esteem and self-love.

NOTE

I am grateful to Arden Rothstein, Ph.D., and Larry Benjamin, Ph.D., who introduced me to clinical neuropsychology and the value of integrating psychoanalytic and neuropsychological perspectives. I am also grateful to the mental health professionals at the Eighteenth Biannual Shaker Mill College Counseling Center Association Meeting (May 1982) who helped clarify my thinking about the role of the diagnostician in the larger university system. I also thank Beth Jung for her secretarial and helpful editorial assistance.

REFERENCES

Alley, G., and Deshler, D. 1979. *Teaching the Learning Disabled Adolescent: Strategies and Methods*. Denver: Love.

Astin, A. W. 1983. *The American Freshman: National Norms for Fall, 1982*. Los Angeles: Laboratory for Research in Higher Education, Graduate School of Education, University of California.

Bellak, L. 1979. Psychiatric aspects of minimal brain dysfunction in adults: their ego function assessment. In L. Bellak, ed. *Psychiatric Aspects of Minimal Brain Dysfunction in Adults*. New York: Grune & Stratton.

Benton, A. L., and Pearl, D. 1978. *Dyslexia: An Appraisal of Current Knowledge*. New York: Oxford University Press.

Clark, F. 1981. *Major Research Findings of the University of Kansas Institute for Research in Learning Disabilities*. Research Report no. 31. Emphasis on Adolescents and Young Adults. Lawrence: Institute for Research in Learning Disabilities, University of Kansas.

Coles, G. S. 1978. The learning disabilities test battery: empirical and social issues. *Harvard Educational Review* 48:313–340.

Crabtree, L. H. 1981. Minimal brain dysfunction in adolescents and young adults: diagnostic and therapeutic perspectives. *Adolescent Psychiatry* 9:307–320.

Cruickshank, W. M.; Morse, W. C.; and Johns, J. S. 1980. *Learning Disabilities: The Struggle from Adolescence toward Adulthood.* Syracuse, N.Y.: Syracuse University Press.

Dinklage, K. T. 1971. Inability to learn a foreign language. In G. Blaine and C. McArthur, eds. *Emotional Problems of the Student.* 2d ed. New York: Appleton-Century-Crofts.

Farnham-Diggory, S. 1980. Learning disabilities: a view from cognitive science. *Journal of the American Academy of Child Psychiatry* 19:570–598.

Fielding, P. M. 1981. *A National Directory of Four-Year Colleges, Two-Year Colleges, and Post High School Training Programs for Young People with Learning Disabilities.* 4th ed. New York: Partners in Publishing.

Frauenheim, J. G. 1978. Academic achievement characteristics of adult males who were diagnosed as dyslexic in childhood. *Journal of Learning Disabilities* 11:476–483.

Gary, R. A. 1981. Services for the LD adult: a working paper. *Learning Disability Quarterly* 4:426–434.

Heinicke, C. M. 1971. Learning disturbances in childhood. In B. B. Wolman, ed. *Manual of Child Psychopathology.* New York: McGraw-Hill.

Horowitz, H. A. 1981. Psychiatric casualties of minimal brain dysfunction in adolescents. *Adolescent Psychiatry* 9:275—294.

Kline, C. C., and Kline, C. L. 1975. Follow-up study of 216 dyslexic children. *Bulletin of the Orton Society* 25:125–144.

Medalie, J. 1981. The college years as a mini-life cycle: developmental tasks and adaptive options. *Journal of the American College Health Association* 30:75–79.

Miller, D. C.; McKinley, D. L.; and Ryan, M. 1979. College students: learning disabilities and services. *Personnel and Guidance Journal* 58:154–158.

Ochroch, R. 1981. A review of the minimal brain dysfunction syndrome. In R. Ochroch, ed. *The Diagnosis and Treatment of Minimal Brain Dysfunction in Children.* New York: Human Sciences.

Pine, F. 1980. On phase-characteristic pathology of the school-age child: disturbances of personality development and organization (borderline conditions), of learning, and of behavior. In S. I. Greenspan and G. H. Pollack, eds. *The Course of Life: Psychoanalytic Contributions toward Understanding Personality Development.* Vol. 2. Washington, D.C.: Government Printing Office.

Rist, R. C., and Harrell, J. E. 1982. Labeling the learning disabled child: the social etiology of educational practice. *American Journal of Orthopsychiatry* 52:146–160.

Rothstein, A. 1982. An integrative perspective on the diagnosis of learning disorders. *Journal of the American Academy of Child Psychiatry* 21:420–426.

Rudel, R. G. 1980. Learning disability: diagnosis by exclusion and discrepancy. *Journal of the American Academy of Child Psychiatry* 19:547–569.

Rudel, R. G. 1981. Residual effects of childhood reading disabilities. *Bulletin of the Orton Society* 31:89–100.

Rutter, M. 1978. Prevalence and types of dyslexia. In A. L. Benton and D. Pearl, eds. *Dyslexia: An Appraisal of Current Knowledge.* New York: Oxford University Press.

Schumaker, J. B.; Deshler, D. D.; Denton, P.; Alley, G. R.; Clark, F. L.; and Warner, M. M. 1981. *Multipass: A Learning Strategy for Improving Reading Comprehension.* Research Report no. 33. Lawrence: Institute for Research in Learning Disabilities, University of Kansas.

Schumaker, J. B.; Deshler, D. D.; Nolan, S.; Clark, F. L.; Alley, G. R.; and Warner, M. M. 1981. *Error Monitoring: A Learning Strategy for Improving Academic Performance of LD Adolescents.* Research Report no. 32. Lawrence: Institute for Research in Learning Disabilities, University of Kansas.

Siegel, E. 1975. *The Exceptional Child Grows Up.* New York: Dutton.

Slack, W. V., and Porter, D. 1980. The Scholastic Aptitude Tests: a critical appraisal. *Harvard Educational Review* 50:154–175.

Weiss, G.; Hechtman, L.; and Pearlman, T. 1978. Hyperactives as young adults: school, employer and self-rating obtained during 10-year follow-up evaluations. *American Journal of Orthopsychiatry* 48:438–445.

14 SEXUAL ABUSE OF CHILDREN AND ADOLESCENTS

MAX SUGAR

That sexual abuse of children occurs with those of varying degree of consanguinity and proximity is still difficult for many people, including professionals, to accept.

"Incest is now coming out of the closet, and one child in every ten families could be a victim of incest. This is often consensual between brothers and sisters, but it may also involve an adult, usually a father, or mother, uncle, etc." (*New Orleans Times-Picayune* 1981). Other sources feel that one out of ten, or more, children are sexually abused, more often not by strangers (Finkelhor 1982; *Newsweek* 1982; Rush 1981). Kempe (1978) believes sexual abuse is "just as common as physical abuse and failure to thrive." Steele (1980) feels that physical and sexual abuse often coexist.

This chapter will examine some clinical and developmental aspects of sexually abused youngsters.

Review of Literature

In 1932, Ferenczi described the confusion of children's tender play with adults' sexual passions, which then are forced on the child. He went on to say (1955, p. 161):

Even children of very respectable, sincerely puritanical families fall victim to real violence or rape much more often than one had dared to suppose. Either it is the parents who try to find a substitute gratification in this pathological way for their frustration, or it is people thought to be trustworthy, such as relatives (uncles, aunts, grandparents), governesses or servants, who misuse the ignorance of the child. The immediate explanation—that these are only sexual fantasies of the child, a kind of hysterical lying—is unfortunately made invalid by the number of such confessions, e.g. of assault upon children, committed by patients actually in analysis. . . . They mistake the play of children for the desires of a sexually mature person or even allow themselves—irrespective of any consequences—to be carried away.

The real rape of girls who have hardly grown out of the age of infants, similar sexual acts of mature women with boys, and also enforced homosexual acts, are more frequent occurrences than had hitherto been assumed.

There are few data from analyses of adults about their feelings or motives related to being involved in inappropriate sleeping arrangements with, or sexual abuse of, children (Ferenczi 1955; Litin, Giffin, and Johnson 1956). This is all the more remarkable since the analytic literature is replete with references to the effects of the primal scene. Ferenczi noted that the child reacts to the sexual intrusion by the adult in ways that would be unexpected; that is, the child tends to minimize it, or feels it is not something that was inflicted on him (or her), or treats it as a fantasy and not as an actuality. He related this to the child's need for identification with the adult as well as the need and wish for acceptance that follows the child's complying with the adult's wishes.

This recalls the findings by Johnson, Giffin, Watson, and Beckett (1956) from collaborative therapy, and those of Beckett, Robinson, Frazier, Steinhilber, Duncan, Estes, Litin, Gratten, Lorton, Williams, and Johnson (1956), who noted that patients' material containing traumatic assaults on them as children occurred frequently; with the use of collaborative therapy, these data were confirmed.

Incest between fathers and daughters has been better documented than mothers' untoward sexual or abusive behavior to their children, both males and females. There are probably at least as many "closet" homosexual mothers as fathers, despite lesser documentation. Homosexual actions, and even rape, take place between father and son or uncle and nephew, and most of them go unreported.

Media stories about incest are usually between an adult male and a younger female, but sexual exploitation takes place between people of all possible combinations of ages, sexes, and consanguinity (Lewis and

Sarrel 1969; Slovenko 1980). In recent years, increased evidence of child abuse, neglect, and failure to thrive, in addition to other less obvious forms of physical and emotional neglect, has been collected. More of these cases confirming Ferenczi's observations should be forthcoming, and to some extent this is occurring (Finkelhor 1982; Katan 1973; Kempe 1978; Lewis and Sarrel 1969; Rush 1981).

Illustrative Cases

It is important to reconstruct and separate the actual events to which the youngsters were subjected (whether treated as children or adults) from the fantasies, wishes, and fears that they have intertwined with the events. This may be useful to us as clinicians to help understand their adaptations and defenses and at the same time to deal with them in a therapeutic context. The following cases by no means exhaust the possible combinations, and even grandmothers and married aunts are not immune.

MOTHERS AND DAUGHTERS

CASE 1

This mother began sleeping with her daughter and son during their latency years, while the father was working nights. After the mother and father divorced, this continued whenever her boyfriend was not home. The children felt left out and quite jealous if they did not sleep with her when her boyfriend was there. When the son was at his father's and the mother's boyfriend was absent, mother and daughter slept together. The mother drank heavily and occasionally was involved in drug usage.

On occasion, she attempted to have homosexual relations with her adolescent daughter. This led the daughter to rupture relations with the mother, move to the paternal home, and marry prematurely.

FATHERS ABUSING SONS

CASE 2

A middle-aged male was convicted of homosexually molesting his latency-aged son, and his son was placed in a state residential home.

The father successfully manipulated the authorities to contravene their judgment and removed his son from the state institution, and they left the state. The youngster, now in early adolescence, ostensibly was staying in a new residential center because of these considerations, but the father was able to visit him during the week and have the son home on weekends.

The divorced father had had three unsuccessful marriages and was hostile to women. The son's view of women was similar to the father's. He wanted to be accepted and loved by his father, since he was the only parent present, but he was angry and distressed about his father's past sexual assaults.

After several weekends at home, they began sleeping in the same bed. Although the father made efforts not to assault his son and the son was frightened to be with the father, homosexual incest recurred.

ABUSE BY SIBLINGS

CASE 3

At seven a boy was inveigled by his early-adolescent brother to engage in homosexual relations and apparently was accepting of this at first. Then it became a regular, forced feature of their relationship. This continued until he was thirteen, when he stopped and became intensely interested in proving he was not homosexual by excessive heterosexual activity.

There was little in the way of separate ego boundaries for the family members or protection of the young from excess stimulations.

He was anxious, suspicious, and angry toward females and males, with severe difficulties in close relationships. He unconsciously manipulated others into rejecting him. He was also insecure in his sexual identity. With girls, he behaved as his brother had to him, forcing himself sexually on them. He had little enjoyment in intercourse, except for his sense of power. He used alcohol and drugs to temper his intense fear of intimate relationships.

CASE 4

A fourteen-year-old was brought to therapy because of his repeated continued hostile behavior in school and at home. He demeaned teachers, in their presence, to his classmates, which led to his expulsion. He provoked his peers on the slightest pretext, having many fights which he usually lost. Since early childhood, he had lied to one parent about the other as well as about siblings.

Two years after the parents divorced, custody was taken from the mother for neglect and granted to the father. Before the change in custody, the mother had been living with a man she later married. The mother and future stepfather had been observed in intercourse by the patient at age twelve. The father and paternal grandmother called the mother a "whore" and "sleaze" in the children's presence. The father was rigid in applying the talion law for infractions. His stepfather had frequently threatened suicide and homicide with guns and fire setting.

Initially, this youngster's disruptive, impulsive behavior came to be understood as related to feelings of fear and rage about abandonment. Later, intense guilt and the wish for punishment came prominently into the therapeutic picture through the transference. In the course of exploring his guilty feelings, he revealed that he treated his sister as his mother had treated him. Then he brought in material about sexually molesting a five-year-old niece and a toddler nephew. At thirteen, the patient forced his sister, five years younger, to undress, attempted intercourse, and repeatedly humiliated and forced her to undress for him so he would become aroused and masturbate. At other times, he often hog-tied her and picked her up with a broomstick under the elbows. In addition, he often bullied and beat her. For all these events, especially the sexual, he expected a harsh, punitive response and unconsciously arranged for it by hostile behavior for which he expected physical retaliation.

ABUSE BY COUSINS AND BABY-SITTERS

CASE 5

When this youngster entered intensive therapy at age fourteen, she had made a serious suicide attempt; contracted gonorrhea; been a runaway; become pregnant and had an abortion; been truant and failed at school; been guilty of repeated auto and auto parts thefts; and had had promiscuous sexual relationships since she was ten. As the family history was unraveled, it became apparent that there was much acting out by her family extending back several generations—alcoholism, compulsive gambling, bisexuality, and sexual abuse.

Her father told her that, if she became pregnant, he would help her to keep a male, but not a female, child. By contrast, the mother would have rejected her totally. Her maternal uncle read pornography magazines in the bathtub for hours with the door open. At times, he had mutual masturbation with his latency-aged son in the bathtub, which was observed by all in the home, including visitors, such as my patient. The uncle attempted to rape her repeatedly, and no protection was available from the mother or other relatives, not even the minimum of restricting visits to his home. The mother and her female friends took the patient barhopping and the mother's boyfriend lied about her age when questioned in bars. Repeatedly, the mother asked the patient's dates if they had had intercourse on their return from an evening out. The patient bullied and mistreated her brother, four years her junior, and overloaded him with her tales of delinquent behavior.

All her life her mother told her that she had been a mistake (at which her father laughed), and that, at birth, she "had been a problem and almost killed" her mother. After several years of therapy, she divulged that a favorite female cousin, about six years her senior, had forced her into homosexual activities at six years of age. When she told her mother, she was not believed. She was programmed to be like her cousin by being told, "You look and act like her" and dressed like her for years. She was first given drugs at age ten by this cousin, then fifteen, who was abusing drugs and bisexual. At age ten, the patient began heterosexual intercourse under the influence of drugs.

CASE 6

At age four, this youngster was sexually abused by his teenage female cousin. Frightened and unwilling to tell his aunt or his mother, he did not reveal this until in intensive therapy, thirteen years later. He also revealed that he had sexually abused female and male preschoolers in his early teens when he was baby-sitting. His mother was routinely and openly sexually seductive and exhibitionistic, especially after his parents divorced. She lost custody shortly after the divorce because of neglect. She compared his penis size expansively with her lover's, on seeing him undressed in mid adolescence. He observed her in intercourse with her boyfriend through the uncurtained living room window at a time she knew he would be over to visit. Further, he knew of her many indiscriminate sexual liaisons.

His identification with hostile females and problems in sexual identity and trust were readily related to early and continued maternal neglect, hostility, and sexual seductiveness. His identification with his mother involved his superego, evasiveness, and control of impulses, especially aggressive ones.

Discussion

The fact that parents will take youngsters of the same sex into bed as a substitute for their spouses deserves more attention than it has previously been given. Currently, about one out of two marriages ends in divorce in the United States. The stepparents (or surrogate parents) that arise from subsequent marriages (or living together, although unmarried, with their children) have to be considered as additional or potential risk factors if the children sleep with their opposite- (or even same-) sexed parents or stepparents. Where there is no blood tie, the barrier against incest is more easily broken.

When a youngster sleeps with his parents, there may be an invitation to regression, if the youngster is past the autistic or anaclitic stage of object relations. This arrangement invites fixation and lack of progress in the development of separation-individuation; promotes anxieties about the child's abilities to control himself (or herself), his sadistic impulses, and his phallic-oedipal concerns; exploits the child for vicarious parental sexual pleasures; and may enhance superego harshness for the post-oedipal child. The child may need to feel less active and less able to master his surroundings because of the need to avoid exposing his knowledge of what the parents are doing. The mother may be sexually abusive, exhibitionistic, stimulating consciously or unconsciously, and provide a sadistic, seductive, provocative image to the youngster. The same applies to the father.

The concept of cumulative trauma (Khan 1963) seems applicable here. Khan focused on the effects of cumulative trauma based on events at the preverbal stage in the relationship between mother and infant that may affect ego and psychosexual development. An unpleasant event occurring between a parent and a child, whether of the same or of the opposite sex, in a sexual act of whatever degree or sort, or the observance of it by the child, will be reacted to and interpreted differently according to the child's age, stage of development, type of involvement with the adults, intelligence, ability to cope with and integrate events, and particular sensitivities. If the act is repetitious, so that the child cannot recover from one upset before the next befalls him, it is particularly significant in terms of the child's response to the trauma and its developmental effects.

The concatenation of a number of distressing events impressing themselves on a child within a short period, at a time when he feels helpless and unable to do anything but submit, leads to the development of emotional trauma with defensive reactions and symptoms of varying severity. Thus, the current increased potential for sexual abuse of children caused by societal changes and its effects on development must be borne in mind, as outlined by Lewis and Sarrel (1969).

Hirsch (1975) wrote of Charles Dickens's nurse stories:

> Throughout all the tales, in fact, the child's helpless passivity is contrasted with the active threats of adults and their zoological surrogates. Dickens insists that even his storytelling nurse seemed to have "a fiendish enjoyment of my terrors," and that, though "her name was Mercy . . . she had none on me. . . ."
>
> These five nurses' stories are in fact variations on or portions of a single fantasy or experience common to infancy and which psychoanalysis calls the primal scene . . . reinforces the hypothesis that these tales ultimately derive from memories or fantasies of watching parental copulation.

Hirsch (1975) assumes that Dickens's stories were an inaccurate rendering of childhood events and only a fantasy.

The observations by Katan (1973) on children who were raped led her to state:

> When Freud found out that his patients' reports about their fathers' seductions of them were fantasies, it led to the discovery of the oedipal conflict. Analyses at that time did not reach the depth they did later. I have often wondered whether these patients of Freud's had not been right about one thing. The sexual seduction or rape that victimized them in early childhood may well have been a reality but was attributed by them to the wrong person, to their fathers.

Perhaps the time to revise some aspects of theory is overdue. If the facts are not separated from the fantasy and the patient's confusion settled, then treatment will be confusing and stalemated. If reality and fantasy are not separated, the therapist is then treating the patient's trauma as a fantasy, which the patient perceives as a dismissal of its actuality or impact, just as the initial perpetrator of the trauma did.

The patients in cases 3, 4, 5, and 6 revealed the material only after lengthy therapy and when at a stage of trust. Earlier in therapy, it was understandably difficult to reveal such data because of the transference expectation of another assault or rejection. Case 5 is especially reflective of the programming effects (Litin et al. 1956) and the problem of a pathological symbiosis.

Any therapy for such assaults would have to begin with their cessation. This requires separating fiction from fact, followed by intervention with the parents or parent surrogates, since it is child abuse. Prevention of bedroom assaults on children should begin with bedroom privacy for them from the parents and other adults as well as opposite-sexed siblings (Sugar 1975). When assaults have occurred, therapy is necessary, since the emotional impact may be searingly deleterious to development (Katan 1973) in childhood and adolescence. Intense guilt about having sexually abused younger children may be the source of an adolescent's suicidal behavior or provocativeness leading to rejection or delinquent acts with unconscious arrangements (which appear to be begging) for apprehension and punishment.

If a patient reveals being sexually abused as a child, then his identification with the aggressor cannot be far behind; and, if therapy continues, material relevant to his inflicting it on others may be expected to be forthcoming.

It seems, from clinical material, that where there is sexual or physical abuse, there is a pathological symbiosis with neglect, and vice versa. A pathological symbiosis involves parental exploitation of the child; role reversal, with the child taking care of parental needs; neglect of the child's needs; blurring of ego boundaries; obstruction to ego differentiation; and overindulgence of the child. This amounts to emotional neglect and abuse by the parent. The degree of emotional and sexual abuse increases in proportion to the degree of consanguinity. Thus, incest involves a pathological symbiosis and neglect.

The neglect and abuse may have begun very early in life, leading to an avoidance-aggressive pattern in response to maternal rejection (ignoring but maintaining physical contact), as described by George and Main (1979) and Wasserman, Green, and Allen (1983).

In the cases presented above, the parents' personality features seem similar to those described for physical child abusers (Steele and Pollock 1968). Even where the parent was not the sexual abuser, that person often was a passive contributor through neglect.

After the youngsters in cases 3, 4, 5, and 6 had been in intensive therapy for a lengthy period, the defensive pattern outlined here emerged with almost routine regularity. They had had some early effects of imprinting and identification with the aggressor toward developing a sadomasochistic and highly distrustful distancing orientation toward all, but especially neglectful maternal figures. They constantly sought, but feared, closeness, intimacy, and caring. However, by their hostility, projection, splitting, and denial, they managed to alienate people. If someone dared to like them, they were suspicious and looked for flaws and slights by which they could promote a physical or verbal battle, ending in distance and separation. If people did not respond immediately and warmly to them, they felt rejected. With confabulation and sabotaging, a patient would arrange for his acquaintances and friends to be suspicious of, or angry at, one another, while the patient felt grandiosely like an orchestra conductor. This ended in a crashing rejection when the exploitation was exposed.

Precocious heterosexual or homosexual relations may be an indicator that the patient was sexually abused. This is all the more so where the sexual relations are devoid of any sense of responsibility or tenderness. In case 4, as well as some of the others, clear-cut hate and revengeful feelings with sadistic behavior were involved in the use of sexuality by the patient for revenge and identification with the aggressor. Features of a posttraumatic stress disorder are present in various combinations with other diagnoses in these cases.

The pattern of trying to master their earlier trauma (of neglect, physical and sexual abuse) by trusted ones was intertwined with identification with the aggressor. The molested youngsters thus became the molesting youngsters, by doing unto others what had been done to them. This is similar to the findings of Steele and co-workers (1968, 1970) that almost all abusing parents have a personal history of deprivation, neglect, or physical abuse in childhood.

Similar ancient observations may have been the stimulus whereby Rabbi Hillel (Pirkei Avot 1967)

> . . . saw a skull floating on the water and said to it ''Because you

have drowned others, they have drowned you and in the end they will be drowned.''

This is in keeping with the observation by Marohn (1982) that a markedly high percentage of delinquent, violent youths die violent deaths. Lewis and co-workers (Lewis, Shanok, Pincus, and Glaser 1979) noted that violent delinquent youngsters have had more physical abuse, illness, and injuries as younger children. We should not be surprised if they were to find that these violent youngsters were also victims of sexual abuse.

Summary

Parents, relatives, and friends may inflict their passions on children of the same or opposite sex. This is often initiated by sleeping together. Sexual abuse contributes to and causes emotional trauma, although the child's turmoil, confusion, wish for acceptance, and anxiety may be overlooked by the parent and professional. Mutual silence aided by threats adds to the anxiety.

Despite the notion that reports of parental sexual exploitation of their children are usually fantasies, there appear to be increasing data that incest and sexual abuse are frequent traumata. At present, there is increased risk of lowering the incest barrier because of increased rates of divorce and step- or surrogate parenthood, since they provide additional potential for being sexually and emotionally traumatized.

Sexual abuse seems to be part of a constellation involving neglect and a pathological symbiosis. That sexual abuse is emotionally traumatic is apparent, but it needs emphasizing. Children's defensive reactions may cloud this, and it may be years before such incidents are connected to symptomatic behavior, even when the child is in intensive therapy. In the reported cases, there appears to be a pattern of reactions and defenses related to the traumata that are embedded in imprinting and identification with the aggressor. This leads to sexual abuse being a legacy passed on to the next generation of victims, as the victim becomes the molester through identification. Adolescent self-destructive behavior may stem from guilt about sexually abusing younger children.

Therapists may be better able to understand and deal with some of their patients' symptoms if sexual abuse is considered as a possible factor in one or both directions.

REFERENCES

Beckett, P. G.; Robinson, D. B.; Frazier, D. H.; Steinhilber, R. M.; Duncan, G. M.; Estes, H. R.; Litin, E. M.; Gratten, R. T.; Lorton, W. L.; Williams, G. E.; and Johnson, A. M. 1956. Studies in schizophrenia at the Mayo Clinic. I. The significance of exogenous traumata in the genesis of schizophrenia. *Psychiatry* 19:137–142.

Ferenczi, S. 1955. Confusion of tongues between adults and the child. In *Final Contributions to the Problems and Methods of Psychoanalysis.* Vol. 3. New York: Basic.

Finkelhor, D. 1982. *Sexually Victimized Children.* New York: Free Press.

George, C., and Main, M. 1979. Social interaction of young abused children: approach, avoidance, and aggression. *Child Development* 50:306–318.

Hirsch, G. D. 1975. Charles Dickens' Nurse Stories. *Psychoanalytic Review* 62:173–179.

Johnson, A. M.; Giffin, M. E.; Watson, E. J.; and Beckett, P. G. 1956. Studies in schizophrenia at the Mayo Clinic. II. Observations on ego functions in schizophrenia. *Psychiatry* 19:143–148.

Katan, A. 1973. Children who were raped. *Psychoanalytic Study of the Child* 28:208–224.

Kempe, C. H. 1978. Sexual abuse, another hidden pediatric problem. *Pediatrics* 62:382–389.

Khan, M. M. R. 1963. The concept of cumulative trauma. *Psychoanalytic Study of the Child* 18:286–306.

Lewis, D. O.; Shanok, S. S.; Pincus, J. H.; and Glaser, G. H. 1979. Violent juvenile delinquents: psychiatric, neurological, psychological, and abuse factors. *Journal of the American Academy of Child Psychiatry* 18:307–319.

Lewis, M., and Sarrel, P. M. 1969. Some psychological aspects of seduction, incest, and rape in childhood. *Journal of the American Academy of Child Psychiatry* 8:606–619.

Litin, E. M.; Giffin, M. E.; and Johnson, A. M. 1956. Parental influence in unusual sexual behavior in children. *Psychoanalytic Quarterly* 25:37–55.

Marohn, R. 1982. Adolescent violence. *Journal of the American Academy of Child Psychiatry* 21:354–360.

New Orleans Times Picayune. 1981. Incest: the secret is being told. November 16.

Newsweek. 1982. Beware of child molesters. August 9.

Pirkei Avot. Ethics of the Talmud: sayings of the fathers—the Mishna 2:7. New York: Schocken, 1967.

Rush, F. 1981. *The Best Kept Secret*. New York: McGraw-Hill.

Slovenko, R. 1980. Criminal laws setting boundaries on sexual exploitation. In M. Sugar, ed. *Responding to Adolescent Needs*. New York: Spectrum.

Steele, B. F. 1970. Parental abuse of infants and small children. In E. J. Anthony and T. Benedek, eds. *Parenthood, Its Psychology and Psychopathology*. Boston: Little, Brown.

Steele, B. F. 1980. Psychodynamic factors in child abuse. In C. H. Kempe and R. E. Helfer, eds. *The Battered Child*. 3d ed. Chicago: University of Chicago Press.

Steele, B. F., and Pollock, C. H. 1968. A psychiatric study of parents who abuse infants and small children. In R. F. Helfer and H. C. Kempe, eds. *The Battered Child*. Chicago: University of Chicago Press.

Sugar, M. 1975. Children's need for bedroom privacy. *Human Sexuality* 9:50–58.

Wasserman, G. A.; Green, A.; and Allen, R. 1983. Going beyond abuse; maladaptive patterns of interaction in abusing mother-infant pairs. *Journal of the American Academy of Child Psychiatry* 22:245–256.

THE AUTHORS

PETER BLOS is a Faculty Member and Supervisor of Child and Adolescent Analysis at the New York Psychoanalytic Institute. He is past President of the American Association for Child Analysis and a recipient of the Distinguished Service Award of the American Society for Adolescent Psychiatry.

LAURIE M. BRANDT is Assistant Attending Psychologist, McLean Hospital, Belmont, Massachusetts.

JONATHAN COHEN is Clinical Psychologist, Columbia College Counseling Service, and Lecturer, Department of Human Development, Columbia University, New York.

RUDOLF EKSTEIN is Senior Faculty Member and Training Analyst, Los Angeles Psychoanalytic Society and Institute and Southern California Psychoanalytic Institute; Clinical Professor of Medical Psychology, University of California, Los Angeles; and Annual Guest Professor at the University of Vienna.

ERIK H. ERIKSON is Professor of Human Development and Lecturer in Psychiatry, Emeritus, Harvard University, Cambridge, Massachusetts.

CARL B. FEINSTEIN is Director, Outpatient Psychiatry, Children's Hospital National Medical Center, and Associate Professor, Department of Psychiatry and Behavioral Sciences, George Washington University, Washington, D. C.

JERRY M. LEWIS is Psychiatrist-in-Chief, Timberlawn Hospital, and Director, Timberlawn Psychiatric Research Foundation, Dallas, Texas.

JOHN G. LOONEY is Child Psychiatrist and Research Psychiatrist, Timberlawn Hospital, Dallas, Texas.

SOL NICHTERN is Director of Psychiatry, Jewish Child Care Association of New York.

DAVID A. ROTHSTEIN is Attending Physician, Michael Reese Hospital Psychosomatic and Psychiatric Institute, and Clinical Associate Professor of Psychiatry, University of Chicago Pritzker School of Medicine, Chicago, Illinois.

ALBERT J. SOLNIT is Sterling Professor of Pediatrics and Psychiatry, School of Medicine, and Director, Child Study Center, Yale University, New Haven, Connecticut.

DEBORAH ANNE SOSIN is Psychiatric Social Worker, Cambridge, Massachusetts.

MICHAEL H. STONE is Professor and Clinical Director, Department of Psychiatry, University of Connecticut Health Center, Farmington, Connecticut.

MAX SUGAR is Clinical Professor of Psychiatry, Louisiana State University Medical Center, and Unit Director of the Children's Unit, Coliseum Medical Center, New Orleans, Louisiana. He is Editor of this volume.

CONTENTS OF VOLUMES I–X

216

217

222

226

230

NAME INDEX

235

SUBJECT INDEX

Academia, 35–60
  case study in, 44–45
  and Freud, 47, 48
  and grandiosity, 53
  and identity formation, 44–48
  as means to maintain narcissistic balance, 48–51
Academia Castellana, 47
Academic difficulty, as first evidence of learning disability, 180
Academic preferences, and learning disability, 181
Academic requirements, and learning disability, 192
Acceptance, children's wish for, and sexual abuse, 200, 202
Achievements, educational, of black and white students, 67–68
Adaptation, capacity for, and reality testing, 19
Adolescence
  as critical stage of development, 14
  developmental tasks of, 18–19, 22
  and parenthood, reflections, 9–12
  and social and cultural change, 16–17
  theories of turmoil and instability, 19–20
Adolescence to parenthood, obstacles in journey, 14–25
Adolescent, psychotic, symptoms of, 138–39
Adolescent deaf boys, 147–59
"Adolescent egocentrism," and the diarist, 93
Adolescent female development, and the diary as transitional object, 92–102
Adolescent patient's environment, regulating, 171–72
Adolescent self, and termination of treatment, 125–45
Adolescents
  borderline, and the fairy tale, 75–90
  borderline, from wealthy families, 163–75
  competent, from different socioeconomic and ethnic contexts, 64–73
  psychotherapy of, 104–24
  sexual abuse of, 199–209
Adoption, and the fantasy family, 31–33

Affect, depressive, 64
Aggression, and deaf boys, 151. *See also* Violence
Agoraphobia, 110–11
  case study of, as symptom, 110–23
Alcohol
  and unresolved conflicts and needs, 18
  use among students, 70
Ambivalence, and diary writing, 100
Analytical process
  different for adults and adolescents, 125–26
  nature of, 132
Anna Freud remembered, 5–8
Anna Freud Kindergarten, 7
Anorexia nervosa, and borderline adolescents, 164
Antipathic emotional attitude, and the threat of nuclear extinction, 12
Antisocial behavior, and wealth, 164, 166
Anxiety
  and optimal psychic functioning, 105
  situational, 64
"Anxiety attacks," related in therapy, 82–83
Apprenticeship, status of, and the army, 57
Army
  and adolescent process, 47–49
  and grandiosity, 53
  and identity formation, 35–60
  and narcissistic balance, 51–53, 58
"As-if" personality, 170
Aspirations, of black and white students, 67–68
Assessment. *See* Diagnosis
Athletic activities, black and white girls' participation in, 68
Attachment behavior, in conflict with separation behavior, 127–28
Attention span, and deaf boys, 151–52
Auditory-related disabilities, and foreign language acquisition, 185
Authority, and black and white students, 70
"Authority confusion," and the army, 58

"Bad mother," as seen in fairy tales, 81

239